# W.K. KELLOGG FOUNDATION

*Mission Statement*
To help people help themselves through
the practical application of knowledge and
resources to improve their quality of life
and that of future generations.

# American Public Health Association

*Mission Statement*
APHA is an association of individuals and organizations working to improve
the public's health. It promotes the scientific and professional foundation of
public health practice and policy, advocates the conditions for a healthy global society,
emphasizes prevention, and enhances the ability of members to promote and
protect environmental and community health.

## Community–Based Public Health:

# A Partnership Model

**Edited by**
**Thomas A. Bruce**
**Steven Uranga McKane**

#45117232

American Public Health Association
800 I Street, N.W.
Washington, DC 20001-3710
http://www.apha.org

Mohammad N. Akhter, MD, MPH
Executive Vice President

2.0M  05/00

Library of Congress Card Number: 00-103145

ISBN: 0-87553-184-9

The use of trade names and commercial sources by authors in certain chapters does not imply endorsement by either APHA or the editorial board of this book.

*Printed and bound in the United States of America.*

*Cover and book design by:* Designworks

*Typeset in:* Bembo and Helvetica

*Printing and Binding:* United Book Press, Inc.

# Contents

# Foreword

*Community-Based Public Health: A Partnership Model* is a timely publication – not only for institutions of public health, but for any institution actively seeking to work with communities. Today, developing meaningful partnerships with the communities they serve is crucial to the success of institutions, nonprofit organizations, and corporations. The material contained in the following pages contributes to a wider understanding of how to initiate and sustain viable partnerships and improve community life in the process.

The Kellogg Foundation's Community-Based Public Health (CBPH) Initiative focused on public health practice in communities, the education and training of public health professionals at colleges and universities, and public health research and scholarly practice within academic institutions. The goal was actively to link education with practice and engage community people in the process of setting the course for public health pursuits in their neighborhoods and communities. During my tenure at Johns Hopkins University, I worked closely with Community-Based Public Health Initiative partners in East Baltimore. We emphasized student learning informed by what was happening in the field of practice – and making the work of academic institutions more relevant to the health challenges of people in communities. In the spirit of this philosophy, public health students' involvement in communities reflected a long-term commitment to public health and serving the community.

Some would suggest that focusing on practice-based learning tends to weaken theoretical and intellectual foundations, and diminish professional education. But I have observed the opposite: significant learning occurs in the context of application. The experiences of Community-Based Public Health Initiative partners underscore this lesson.

The public health institutions of today function in a world their founders would barely recognize. Expanding globalization spurs the need for multicultural competencies. New market forces require sophisticated skills in management. Unprecedented access to information creates an ongoing pressure to collect, analyze, store, and index data. Public policies devolving responsibility for service delivery and economic development to local agencies are redirecting funding and programming at the community level. As public health institutions strive to address new demands and capitalize on opportunities, innovative approaches will be critical to their ultimate success.

*Creating a vision, setting an agenda, building coalitions, maintaining viable partnerships – Community-Based Public Health grantees have these lessons to share for the future of public health.*

Creating a vision, setting an agenda, building coalitions, maintaining viable partnerships – Community-Based Public Health grantees have these lessons to share for the future of public health. Community-Based Public Health experiences also illustrate the role of the policy process in improving health and fostering community development. Philanthropic organizations can engender models and expand societal options for solving complex problems. But ultimately, CBPH partners and Kellogg Foundation grantees remind us, the process of reshaping public health systems must be supported at many levels within the public and private sectors.

**William C. Richardson, Ph.D.**
*President and CEO*
W.K. Kellogg Foundation

iii

iv

# Preface

A basic tenet of W.K. Kellogg Foundation programming is the belief that communities, health practitioners, and academicians working together hold the greatest promise for improving the health and well-being of people. Yet health systems in the United States seem to be growing more fragmented, not less so, even as the unmet health and human service needs of people remain considerable. And the public health profession – which is responsible for assuring community conditions that promote health – often has neither the resources nor the personnel to help shape health systems to better meet community needs.

Lamentably, and in spite of some notable successes, the American health care system has all too frequently been unable to realize its potential to improve the health of the public. Public health programs are commonly underfunded and understaffed, limited by a paucity of trained personnel, often overwhelmed by the demand for direct care services, and perceived by some to be mired in politics and drowning in bureaucracy. Under the circumstances, the profession has altogether too few leaders at the local level with the vision and skills needed to revitalize public health agencies for a new era.

However, the pressures of the health care marketplace and the related demands of a changing society may present an opportunity to reconfigure and strengthen a public health system sorely in need of attention.

Public health's unique focus through the years has been on prevention strategies that target entire communities, in contrast to the health care system's focus on delivery of services to individuals. At a time when the costs for illness care are rising, and the health care marketplace is driving the forces of change, new approaches that emphasize prevention over cure attract particular interest.

The nature of societal health issues also is shifting. When great epidemics threatened the populace, public health sent teams of epidemiologists and infectious disease experts into besieged communities to identify and launch an attack on the offending agents. But these approaches seem less relevant to today's public health challenges – things like violence, substance abuse, and chronic diseases that result from longstanding biopsychosocial and behavioral problems. These complex societal challenges cry out for more diligent efforts to create solid public-private partnerships, multiagency coalitions, and comprehensive community-based responses.

In 1988 the Institute of Medicine (IOM) at the National Academy of Sciences studied and made recommendations on these issues in *The Future of Public Health*. This report, supported in part by the W.K. Kellogg Foundation, provided a clarion call to recognize and address issues facing the profession and set in motion many of the events which led to the genesis of the Community-Based Public Health Initiative.

To lend credence to public health approaches as a valid way for improving the overall health system, the Kellogg Foundation in 1990 elected to support an IOM recommendation that the education and training of public health students be made more relevant to practice within the field. The Foundation's perspective, based upon decades of experience with grantees working in local communities, was that education should be linked not only with the realities of public health practice, but with the day-to-day experiences of people in communities who struggle firsthand with public health challenges.

Kellogg Foundation program leaders believed that public health graduates of the future would best be able to provide genuine leadership if they mastered not only traditional disciplines (epidemiology, biostatistics, environmental health, and health services administration), but also an understanding of the people being served. Such understanding would come not from being taught *about* the community, but from working *with* the community and learning directly about issues and practical, promising approaches to improving health. One crucial dimension of this approach was bringing public health into the mainstream of each community's health service sector, thus avoiding the isolationist role it too often assumed among the other health professions.

In January 1991, the Kellogg Foundation announced the **Community-Based Public Health (CBPH) Initiative**. Its aim was to strengthen the practice and teaching of public health by creating partnerships with an informed and involved public. Models were to be based in underserved communities in the United States, and the people who lived in those communities were to share responsibility and ownership in the work of public health.

The initiative was simple in concept, but complex in the way it was implemented. A consortium or community/agency partnership was at the core of the CBPH strategy to achieve project goals. Over the five-year grant period most CBPH objectives were realized in spite of some major challenges, and consortium partners learned a great deal in the process. The single most important lesson emerging from the CBPH Initiative was that a community-based approach to public health education and training was not only feasible, but could be transforming in its impact on students, faculty, the educational process, and the culture of academic institutions. A secondary lesson, judging from indicators, was that community-based approaches resulted in stronger community health agencies and healthier communities.

This book has been compiled to share information – on contextual issues, the CBPH vision, strategies and approaches, stakeholders engaged in the process, and benchmarks and desired outcomes – with others interested in improving community health by developing working consortiums. The eleven chapters, along with appendices and references, have been compiled to assist leaders in academic institutions, public health agencies, health systems, and community organizations in both appreciating the scope of the CBPH undertaking and drawing from it lessons to inform their related pursuits.

The first three chapters are an overview of the history, context, and philosophical underpinnings of the CBPH Initiative. Chapter I details a historical outline and chronology for the initiative. In Chapter II, John McKnight describes a philosophy that places ordinary citizens at the center of efforts to address complex societal issues. In Chapter III, Dalton Paxman, Philip Lee, and David Satcher discuss the achievements and challenges of the public health profession at the beginning of the twenty-first century.

Chapters IV through VII provide the perspectives of consortium partners – community organizations, academic groups, and practice agencies. In Chapter IV, Quinton Baker, a community representative during the CBPH Initiative, gives his perspective on the relevance and significance of community engagement. Chapters V and VI analyze academic perspectives. In Chapter V, members of the North Carolina consortium speak to the educational changes that resulted from CBPH. In Chapter VI, members of the Michigan consortium

describe the very different way research is carried out when community people become active partners. And in Chapter VII, Robert Pestronk details the approach he took as public health director in linking with community organizations and academic partners to address health needs in his own Michigan community.

Chapters VIII through X focus on some key elements of the CBPH Integrated Action Plan – a planning tool for linking evaluation, communication, and policy work. In Chapter VIII, Toby Citrin, who provided support for the CBPH Initiative's National Policy Task Force, details the process involved in addressing the policy implications of community-based efforts. In Chapter IX, Connie Schmitz, director of the CBPH Cluster Evaluation Team, reviews what was learned through the CBPH Initiative and examines related costs. And Chapter X looks at the overall significance of the community-based approach in terms of public health.

In the final chapter, Gloria Smith, W.K. Kellogg Foundation Vice President for Programs – Health, and Kay Randolph-Back, Program Analyst, examine the history, concepts, and accomplishments of CBPH within the context of changes in philanthropy and society.

It is our hope that public health faculty and practitioners, researchers, colleagues in philanthropy, and leaders of community-based organizations will find this volume a useful one. It represents the dedication and diligence of hundreds of students, teachers, public health workers, and community members – the people who made the CBPH Initiative an invaluable experience. Their communities and institutions are stronger because of their spirited resolve and participation. By sharing the lessons from their collective work, we hope other communities and institutions will reap the same benefits.

*The single most important lesson emerging from the CBPH Initiative was that a community-based approach to public health education and training was not only feasible, but could be transforming in its impact on students, faculty, the educational process, and the culture of academic institutions.*

**Thomas A. Bruce**
Little Rock, Arkansas


**Steven Uranga McKane**
Woodland Hills, California

# Acknowledgments

This book was made possible because thousands of people from across the United States came together during the early 1990s to participate in a bold new venture for health improvement. What made the effort so notable was not the attempt to build coalitions to advance a worthy cause or to explore new approaches to collaboration, although these clearly were of value. It also was not because of the urgent need to try new ways to address the social and behavioral causes of premature death in our society, though that too was a consideration. The remarkable thing about the Community-Based Public Health (CBPH) Initiative was that it brought together such vastly different players into concerted action. If ever there was an "unnatural marriage," this was it. On the one hand were the teachers, investigators, and practitioners in one of the oldest health professions. On the other were people in communities – some struggling to make ends meet, many with little knowledge about the way the health system works and little desire to master it. Indeed, if there was anything the two groups had in common at the outset of the CBPH Initiative it was their skepticism about working cooperatively towards a common goal.

But they did it, and to all who made the commitment we owe our special thanks. Within a year of starting the process, thrown together in the crucible of experimental learning, participants moved from tolerance, to respect, to collegiality, and to genuine admiration for one another. This unholy union gave birth to the lessons reported in this book.

Two Kellogg Foundation senior officers have our heartfelt thanks for their foresight and leadership in starting and carrying through the CBPH Initiative. Dr. Helen K. Grace was the Vice President for Health Programs at the outset, and of all those involved she had the clearest vision of the role that community people can play in pushing for health improvements and advocating for health institutional reform. Her successor, Dr. Gloria R. Smith, a former state health department director and a nursing school dean, brought enormous insight to her role, and practical guidance in addressing the challenges of educating and preparing the next generation of public health practitioners.

From the beginning of the initiative, the W.K. Kellogg Foundation Board of Trustees and its Chairman and CEO, Dr. Russell Mawby, were interested and supportive of the project and remained so throughout its course. Midway through the CBPH Initiative, the Board spent a week visiting three of the CBPH sites. They became quite knowledgeable about the fundamental shift in thinking the CBPH Initiative required – especially the shift in responsibility from health professionals to the people in communities. Dr. Mawby's successor as Kellogg Foundation Chairman and CEO, Dr. William C. Richardson, had been deeply involved in the CBPH Baltimore project while serving as President of Johns Hopkins University. He brought his knowledge of the initiative and enthusiasm with him to the Foundation, and provided exemplary leadership in the final years of CBPH. We are most appreciative of the encouragement and support of both of these phenomenal men.

It would have been impossible to mount such a large national initiative without the support of our staff colleagues at the Kellogg Foundation. They helped review proposals, made site visits, and participated actively in strategic planning during all phases of the work. We would like to recognize the following with genuine gratitude: Robert DeVries, Gloria Meert, Ronald Richards, and Henrie Treadwell. Kay Randolph-Back helped enormously with sharpening our ideas and messages. Other staff members who were especially helpful included Robin Leonard, Annette Beecham, and Merilyn Burgess. Four senior staff persons provided innumerable hours of support in developing an Integrated Action Plan: Pat Babcock, Jonathan Miller, Tom Reis, and Ricardo Millett. Another Foundation staff member who deserves especially vigorous applause is Roslyn McCallister Brock. She was a core member of the planning and implementation team, a regular participant in all the network meetings, and an ardent promoter of the CBPH philosophy.

Our understanding of what happened during the course of the CBPH Initiative was aided enormously because of the efforts of the Cluster Evaluation Team. Connie Schmitz, who headed that group, continuously challenged us to be more specific in both our questions and in the planned interventions. Her loyalty to the project and sense of responsibility to the participants led her to value confidentiality as a first-order trait, and the quality of her work brought distinction to her profession as well as a large measure of objectivity and integrity to the assessment process.

Marie Warner was a consultant who helped in developing the central communications plan for the initiative. She also worked with the local project directors to develop consortium plans for communicating their own results to key stakeholders. The Foundation's Marketing and Communications unit was also helpful, and we acknowledge our gratitude to Karen Lake and Halcyon Liew in particular.

Positive relationships with leaders in the field were some of the most rewarding aspects of the CBPH Initiative. Although too numerous to be listed here, they include project-level directors, project evaluators, members of the Leadership and Model Development Steering Committee, Program Committees for each of the network meetings, and several task forces – particularly the National Policy Task Force that contributed so mightily during the last year of the initiative. We are no less grateful to those individuals who served through the day-to-day teaching, service, research, and administration of the CBPH Initiative. Many of these were community volunteers who made unbelievable and sustained contributions, and without whom this effort would have been shallow indeed.

Finally, we would like to thank our families for their love and support during all the nights and weekends when we were distracted by duties or were away from home. We apologize for being absent during birthdays and other important family gatherings, and promise NEVER to do it again!

The article by John McKnight that appears as Chapter II in this volume has previously been published under the title "Two Tools for Well-Being." Professor McKnight owns the copyright and has given permission to republish the material here since it provides the theoretical grounding for so much of the CBPH community work.

The article by Lewis H. Margolis and coworkers, written for this book and published here as Chapter V, has been submitted to the *Journal of Community Practice* with the understanding that this book has primary rights to its information.

The article by Amy J. Schulz and coworkers which appears here as Chapter VI was published in the *Journal of Community Practice* in June 1998, and is reprinted here with the express permission of the authors and the *Journal's* editors.

The Johns Hopkins University owns the copyright to the CBPH competencies paper, published here in Appendix A, which has been included in this volume with the consent of the contributing team and the University.

**Thomas A. Bruce**

**Steven Uranga McKane**

viii

# The Authors

**Alice Ammerman, Dr.P.H.,** is Associate Professor, Department of Nutrition, School of Public Health, University of North Carolina at Chapel Hill.

**Quinton E. Baker** is Executive Director of the Center for the Advancement of Community Based Public Health in Durham, North Carolina.

**Irene S. Bayer, M.P.H.,** is a Project Associate with the Office of Community-Based Public Health at the University of Michigan's School of Public Health in Ann Arbor.

**Roslyn McCallister Brock, M.B.A.,** is a Program Associate with the W.K. Kellogg Foundation.

**Thomas A. Bruce, M.D.,** is Professor Emeritus of Medicine at the University of Arkansas for Medical Sciences and a Program Consultant with the W.K. Kellogg Foundation.

**Toby Citrin, J.D.,** is Professor of Public Health and Director of the Office of Community-Based Public Health at the School of Public Health, University of Michigan, Ann Arbor.

**Janice Dodds, Ed.D.,** is an Associate Professor in the Departments of Nutrition and Maternal and Child Health, School of Public Health, University of North Carolina at Chapel Hill.

**Eugenia Eng, Dr.P.H.,** is Associate Professor, Department of Health Behavior and Health Education, School of Public Health, University of North Carolina at Chapel Hill.

**C.B. Griffin** is the former Director of the Community-Based Public Health Project at Agape House, Hartford Memorial Baptist Church, Detroit, Michigan.

**Chris Harlan, M.A., R.N.,** is Research Instructor, Public Health Leadership Program, School of Public Health, University of North Carolina at Chapel Hill.

**Barbara A. Israel, Dr.P.H.,** is Professor and Chair, Department of Health Behavior and Health Education, School of Public Health, University of Michigan, Ann Arbor.

**Barbara Laraia, M.P.H., R.D.,** is a doctoral student, Department of Nutrition, School of Public Health, University of North Carolina at Chapel Hill.

**Philip R. Lee, M.D.,** is a member of the Institute of Health Policy Studies at the University of California in San Francisco and formerly Assistant Secretary for Health, U.S. Department of Health and Human Services.

**Lewis H. Margolis, M.D.,** is Associate Professor of Maternal and Child Health, School of Public Health, University of North Carolina at Chapel Hill.

**Steven Uranga McKane, D.M.D.,** is a private consultant in philanthropy, public health dentistry, and public health management based in Woodland Hills, California.

**John L. McKnight** is Professor of Communication Studies and Urban Affairs and Director of the Program in Community Studies at the Institute for Policy Research, Northwestern University, Evanston, Illinois.

**Dalton G. Paxman, Ph.D.,** is Senior Environmental Health Advisor, Office of Disease Prevention and Health Promotion, U.S. Department of Health and Human Services in Washington, D.C.

**Robert M. Pestronk, M.P.H.,** is Health Officer for Genesee County, Michigan.

**Margaret Pollard, M.P.H.,** is a County Commissioner in Chatham County, North Carolina, and former Director of Public Health and Wellness at the Wake Area Health Education Center, Raleigh, North Carolina.

**Kay Randolph-Back, M.A., J.D.**, is a Program Analyst with the W.K. Kellogg Foundation in Battle Creek, Michigan.

**David Satcher, M.D., Ph.D.**, is Assistant Secretary for Health and Surgeon General, U.S. Department of Health and Human Services, Washington, D.C.

**Connie C. Schmitz, Ph.D.**, is the owner of Professional Evaluation Services, a private consulting firm in Minneapolis, Minnesota, and served as director of the CBPH Cluster Evaluation Team while on staff at the Center for Urban and Regional Affairs, Hubert Humphrey Center, University of Minnesota.

**Amy J. Schulz, Ph.D.**, is Assistant Research Scientist, Department of Health Behavior and Health Education at the School of Public Health, University of Michigan, Ann Arbor.

**Suzanne M. Selig, Ph.D.**, is Professor of Health Care, School of Health Professions and Studies, University of Michigan-Flint.

**Gloria R. Smith, R.N., Ph.D., M.P.H., F.A.A.N.**, is Vice President for Programs - Health at the W.K. Kellogg Foundation in Battle Creek, Michigan.

**Rachel H. Stevens, R.N., Ed.D.**, is Clinical Professor and Director of the Center for Public Health Practice in the School of Public Health, University of North Carolina at Chapel Hill.

# Chapter 1 | History of the Community-Based Public Health Initiative

*Thomas A. Bruce*

The universe of "health" falls into two camps: health care for *individuals* and the health of the *community*. The former usually falls under the aegis of professional caregiver groups and institutions such as hospitals and clinics, and the latter under the public health agencies. The health *care* system typically focuses on medical, nursing, and dental services, whereas the *public* health system more commonly addresses issues related to health promotion and disease prevention. Although there have been repeated attempts to connect these two poles into a unified structure – efforts even now increasing – no real merger has been attained.

Certainly both groups have tried to strengthen connections with the individuals and communities they serve. For decades the concept of "doctor-patient relationship" has been the subject of research to determine ways to improve communication between the professional caregiver and those who receive services. In like manner, the word "public" in public health has been the subject of considerable scrutiny, with the goal of improving outcomes from health campaigns conducted by public agencies. However, viable partnerships based on equity between health professionals and their "customers" have rarely been undertaken, and there is little understanding of the process or the potential value of such an arrangement.

Since its inception, the W.K. Kellogg Foundation has invested in communities to improve the health of people. The Foundation's early work focused on improving access to care, strengthening health care systems, and expanding system capacity to address community health issues. In recent decades, the Kellogg Foundation has initiated and piloted promising models for connecting the resources of health systems with the needs and interests of communities. In 1990, the Foundation announced the Community Partnerships with Health Professions Education Initiative, a multiyear funding effort to redirect the education of health professionals through out-of-hospital training, multidisciplinary education, and community-driven research. The goal was to link communities with academic health centers through formal partnerships. And, although many academic health centers responded to the call for proposals, most included only schools of medicine and nursing in their proposals. Public health programs were largely excluded from the proposed partnerships.

Thus Kellogg Foundation program leaders conceived a parallel initiative to focus on the public health workforce. Drawing on recommendations from the Institute of Medicine's *The Future of Public Health* report, the Community-Based Public Health (CBPH) Initiative was designed to link public health practice and education. In January 1991, the Foundation invited applications from consortia that included both academic programs and public health agencies. Community-based organizations – groups representing people with personal experience related to public health problems – were to be a third key partner. And to address the traditional separation of the public health profession from its clinical disciplines, a fourth partner was required – a health professions school *other* than public health. With the inclusion of these four key stakeholder groups, CBPH was designed to revamp public health education and practice by developing vital partnerships with community-based organizations whose members brought not only health issues to the table, but special strengths and firsthand knowledge of public health systems.

*CBPH was designed to revamp public health education and practice by developing vital partnerships with community-based organizations whose members brought not only health issues to the table, but special strengths and firsthand knowledge of public health systems.*

Announcements were mailed to U.S. universities and their programs of public health, local public health agencies, national and local community-based organizations, and selected Kellogg Foundation grantees. By April 1991, 108 applications had been received. From this group 15 consortia were selected for the planning phase of the project. These semifinalists were invited to participate in a second round of exploration – a year-long leadership and model development phase with reapplication for a four-year CBPH grant at the end of the year.

## The Leadership and Model Development Year

An initial planning period was an important and productive part of the CBPH Initiative. Five seminars were held from September 1991 through March 1992. The information, conceptual development, engagement, and synergy that grew from the five meetings sparked the CBPH implementation phase. The following listing of seminar activities is intended to suggest the conceptual scope of the initiative's development. For more information about how this early work at the national level shaped state and local thinking and implementation, please see Chapters X and XI and Appendix B for related publications.

*Seminar One: Chicago, September 1991* Community, academic, and practice representatives of the 15 consortia met for three days to discuss the tasks ahead. Many chief executive officers, invited for a single day, found the session worthwhile enough that they stayed longer. But it was apparent after the first day's meeting that a great deal of preliminary work would be needed to move the project forward. Most community representatives were unfamiliar with public health and had little idea of why they were included in the initiative. Educators and practice representatives, many of whom were involved in developing the proposals, understood why they were attending, but were unsure about the role community representatives would play. Differences in perspectives among groups were particularly obvious in small group discussions.

One objective of the meeting was to explore the role of community representatives in the consortia. Attendees first learned about the Foundation's programming perspective, then spent an afternoon reviewing and discussing a related case study on the Codman Square Health Center in Boston. The purpose of this exercise was to probe the dimensions of health and community development in an underserved city neighborhood during the course of a Kellogg Foundation grant. In this instance, paraprofessional health workers not only engaged neighborhood residents in health-related activities, but undertook initiatives in economic and housing development, get-

acquainted block parties for social development, and other nontraditional health promotion activities.

On the second day of the seminar, John McKnight of Northwestern University (please see Chapter II) discussed the ways in which a system designed for control can support and nurture community, with all its unique assets and capacities. He touched on community vulnerability and its subversion by training, employment, management – and also addressed volunteerism, citizen participation, and outreach. Following the presentation, a panel of grantees from Kellogg Foundation projects presented the perspectives of African American, Native American, and Latino-Hispanic populations engaged in community-building activities.

At the close of the meeting each consortium met to discuss consortia work plans. Constituency groups (academic, practice, community) also elected representatives to serve on a program steering committee that would operate throughout the Leadership and Model Development phase.

Evaluations of the first seminar indicated that community representatives in particular valued the case study work, but academic and practice representatives were less engaged and worried that the Foundation expected them to pattern their efforts after the Codman Square example. Some academic representatives also felt "bashed" by participants who were critical of university relationships in communities. Individual consortia very much wanted to share their proposed plans and were disappointed at the suggestion that they might need to develop more collaborative approaches.

*Seminar Two: Memphis, October 1991* The three and one-half day session focused on the challenges of public health practice. Speakers reviewed programs of the previous decade, including public health core functions; *Healthy People 2000*; *Healthy Communities: Model Standards*; *Assessment Protocol Excellence in Public Health* (APEX-PH); and CDC's *Planned Approach to Community Health* (PATCH). Content and discussion focused on the potential for linkages between public health agencies, community, and academic partners. Participants also led three panel discussions and engaged in several large and small group discussions. An interactive work session on conflict management was held at the request of participants, and site visits were made to Kellogg Foundation projects in the City of Memphis and in neighboring Mississippi and Arkansas. As in the previous meeting, time was budgeted for consortium groups to meet and work on their proposals.

Evaluation of the second session showed greater cohesion among participants and less competition between consortia groups. The local site visits were particularly helpful in raising the visibility and perceived value of grassroots efforts. Finally, there was the beginning of real synergy from being part of a professionally and ethnically diverse group – one working together for common goals.

*Seminar Three: Atlanta, January 1992* The third conference was electric, full of energy, and the groups seemed to be running, not walking, towards the May due date for complete proposals. The theme of the seminar was the academic role in CBPH. The keynote speaker, Marilyn Aguirre-Molina from the University of Medicine and Dentistry of New Jersey, speculated about the new skills and competencies that public health graduates of the future would need. In addition to the traditional knowledge base (epidemiology, biostatistics, and so on), she concluded there would be major need for (1) community development skills, (2) cross-cultural competency, and (3) a break from a patriarchal/authoritarian mindset. Other presentations during the seminar focused on the Public Health Faculty/Agency Forum recommendations for core public health competencies and the innovative approach to competency-based education under way for several years at Alverno College in Milwaukee. Participants made trips to the Epidemiologic Intelligence Service of the Centers for Disease Control, and to the Carter Presidential Center. Films were shown on the life of W.K. Kellogg and on a model community development project in South Africa. An emotionally powerful presentation was made by the National Black Women's Health project in Atlanta, demonstrating once again the value of community voices in health improvement. Time for individual consortium meetings and constituent group meetings was included in the agenda.

Evaluation of the third session indicated that diversity and trust were being discussed as cross-cutting themes in every group. There was underlying anxiety about the competitive application process, and considerable speculation about the proper balance between cooperation and competition. And, although many positive comments were made about the value of the small group sessions, participants expressed a growing skepticism about the effectiveness of lectures (lectures by university representatives in particular) and of large group discussions often dominated by a few individuals.

*Seminar Four: El Paso, TX, February 1992* The three and one-half day seminar focused on leadership development and governance issues. Participants were given preconference reading assignments of some of John Gardner's articles on leadership. A panel discussion on leadership-in-place was provided by a university president, medical and nursing school deans, the director of a border public health agency, and the director of an award-winning community health center. Site visits were made to two *colonias* on the U.S. side of the border and to some nongovernmental health clinics in Juarez, Mexico, to examine the role of grassroots leadership. Roundtable discussion groups were offered on street approaches to community development, financial development, evaluation planning, institutional change, and the relationship between public health and primary care.

Evaluation of the seminar suggested that pressures were beginning to build within the individual consortia over details related to finalizing the proposal. But participants felt that having individuals come together from vastly different educational, experiential, and cultural backgrounds was a leavening influence that created personal bonds and commitment to a common purpose. This camaraderie was heightened by group travel experiences and by the exhilaration of learning in new settings.

*Seminar Five: Detroit, March 1992* CEOs attended the final seminar to learn more about the initiative as a whole, work with their respective consortia in small group sessions, and collectively brainstorm ways to support the initiative. Participants heard a challenge from Kellogg Foundation CEO Russell Mawby and from Robert Bellah, a prominent sociologist from the University of California at Berkeley, who spoke about the need for greater institutional responsibility in building "The Good Society." A highlight of the session was a celebratory dinner that featured a roast of staff leaders.

Evaluations from the final session reflected the view that the Leadership and Model Development seminar series had been successful from the standpoint of the participants' professional and personal development. People were challenged, changed, and grew individually and collectively in many positive ways. They showed gains in content areas such as team-building skills, knowledge of public health, values and beliefs about diversity and community, and conflict resolution. Whether the seminar series had been powerful enough to create consortia that would survive and thrive over the coming years remained to be seen. But the five seminars represented a promising basis for consortia work to begin the process of revamping public health education and practice, and of developing model approaches to address and improve the public's health at the local level.

3

# Implementation Phase of the Initiative

All 15 consortia participating in the Leadership and Model Development phase submitted full proposals for consideration. A special review panel from within the Foundation assessed the proposals and presented them to the Board of Trustees. Seven were approved for full funding. The remaining eight were offered opportunities to submit mini-grant requests to carry out one or more aspects of their proposals.

---

The seven models of community-based public health were selected on the basis that they offered the best opportunity for successful demonstrations to:

1. **Reorient public health education and practice, programs, and services toward community needs and concerns;**

2. **Ensure that community voices would play a key role by harnessing their assets to partner with professional health leaders and their institutions; and**

3. **Shape a new and more effective health services system, one with a full complement of health promotion and disease prevention approaches for the entire population at each of the local project sites.**

---

The proposals selected were from seven states, and each received funding in September 1992. Individual awards ranged from $1.4 million to $2.24 million over four years. The University of Minnesota was selected to conduct an independent evaluation of the initiative and provide modest technical assistance to project evaluators working in the field.

## The Seven CBPH Projects

The **California** consortium, including community-based organizations located in the East 14th Street Crossroads section of the City of Oakland; the Alameda County Health Care Services Agency; and the University of California Berkeley School of Public Health in conjunction with the University of California San Francisco School of Medicine.

The **Georgia** consortium, including community-based organizations in Cobb County (Rose Garden Hills and Kennesaw Village) and in the University-John Hope Homes public housing units in Atlanta; Cobb County Board of Health; Fulton County Health Department; Emory University Rollins School of Public Health; and the Department of Preventive Medicine at the Morehouse School of Medicine.

The **Maryland** consortium, including Clergy United for Renewal of East Baltimore; Heart, Body & Soul, Inc.; Collington Square, Inc.; Health Care for the Homeless; the Johns Hopkins University Schools of Hygiene and Public Health, Nursing, and Medicine; the Johns Hopkins Hospital; Baltimore City Health Department; and the Baltimore City Public Schools.

The **Massachusetts** consortium, including four community-based coalitions located in central and western Massachusetts (Athol/Orange, Holyoke, Northern Berkshires, and Worcester); the Massachusetts Association of Health Boards; the Area Health Education Centers/Community Partners; the University of Massachusetts School of Public Health; and the University of Massachusetts School of Medicine and its Department of Family Medicine.

The **Michigan** consortium, including Agape House of Hartford Memorial Baptist Church in the City of Detroit; other community-based organizations in Detroit and the City of Flint; the Detroit Health Department; the Genesee County Health Department; the University of Michigan Schools of Public Health and Social Work; University of Michigan-Flint; Wayne State University School of Social Work; and the University of Detroit-Mercy.

The **North Carolina** consortium, including Joint Orange-Chatham Community Action Agency; Strengthening the Black Family, Inc.; Wake Area Health Education Center; the local health departments in Chatham County, Lee County, Orange County, and Wake County; Orange-Chatham Comprehensive Health Services; Wake Health Services; and the University of North Carolina at Chapel Hill Schools of Public Health and Medicine.

The **Washington** consortium, including Garfield Partners in Health; Rainier Partners in Health; the Lummi Indian Nation; the Seattle-King County and Whatcom County Health Departments; Group Health Cooperative of Puget Sound; Northwest Indian College; Seattle Indian Health Board; and the University of Washington Schools of Nursing and Public Health & Community Medicine.

---

**Expected Outcomes:**

1. Teaching, service, and research would more fully reflect the new public health priorities, including community and human development and respect for diversity and pluralism.

2. Core public health functions (assessment, policy development, and assurance) would be performed throughout the initiative in conjunction with the community.

3. All involved organizations would become mission-driven.

4. Multicultural competency would be realized among students, faculty, agency personnel, and community members.

5. Broader participation of people of color in issues of the public's health would be pursued by promoting health and health-related careers in minority populations.

6. Public health values and approaches would be taught/learned in community decision making.

7. More young people would enter public health careers or engage in life work in other helping professions.

8. The models developed would be functional and sustainable.

## Individual Consortium Goals

In addition to the goals and expectations defined for the initiative as a whole, each consortium had its own set of goals. These were spelled out in the initial applications, and reflected in each group's locale, target issues, and partners. Although specific objectives and methods changed as the work progressed, goals for each group's work were articulated at the outset.

The **California** consortium wanted to improve the health and well-being of its targeted community, the East 14th Street Crossroads section of Oakland. The low-income population of 62,583 included several neighborhoods near the Bay Area docks. Many resi-

dents were new immigrants, and the community was in general a highly diverse one, with 41 percent African American, 20 percent Asian, 33 percent Hispanic, and a relatively small but active group of Native American residents. Their plan was to develop a Community Health Academy to provide health education, training, and employment for community residents while offering courses and programs on community development and cultural training for university faculty and students, as well as for health department personnel. They also planned a number of community health campaigns and initiatives, and hoped to offer a variety of other supportive services and professional programs to enhance the local partnership.

A particular strength of the Academy at the outset was its capacity to build multicultural competency and concepts of human/community development among the consortium's partners. Its faculty was drawn from all its collaborating organizations, and it capitalized on the cultural and ethnic diversity of the targeted community and the practical experiences of its grassroots organizations. The faculty members were to serve as leaders in transforming public health education and practice. To facilitate recruitment of community youth into the helping professions, community-based education and mentoring was to be provided by academic and practicing public health professionals, but with liberal use of community individuals and agencies in the programs offered.

The **Georgia** consortium goal was to develop and implement a replicable model of public health practice as a true partnership between the academic institutions, local health departments, and the three targeted communities in the metropolitan Atlanta area. Their plan was to sustain the partnership by employing an empowerment process, using the resources and expertise of the lead institutions to provide the kinds of preventive health services and professional support that would be needed to address community problems and priorities. They wanted to change the way the affiliated institutions thought about their tasks and societal mission. Both Emory and Morehouse saw an opportunity to bridge the gap between theory and practice, and to connect these to community teaching and service.

The **Maryland** consortium hoped to organize a viable consortium in the impoverished and predominantly African-American East Baltimore area. The goal was to foster broad community participation and join academic and practice partners in designing a community

5

prevention program. Neighborhood health workers were to perform screening, outreach, case management, health education, monitoring, and advocacy. A curriculum in community-based public health was to be developed and implemented in the schools of public health, nursing, and medicine, and multidisciplinary practice courses and internships were to be provided in community organizations and health departments. Workshops in health and homelessness were planned annually, and youth health career programs were to cover grades 7-12.

The **Massachusetts** consortium hoped to improve public health within underserved communities in Western Massachusetts through the development of partnerships between communities, public health professionals, and university faculty and students. Through their partnerships they hoped to create new models for learning, strengthen local health agencies, and address fundamental public health problems. They especially wanted to target two representative populations – blue-collar groups living in semirural, economically depressed mill towns, and Latinos living in urban centers – to help them solve their own health problems through joint projects with other consortium partners.

Within the School of Public Health, they hoped to establish an innovative, multicultural, community-based approach to the preparation of public health professionals. They also wanted to promote the capacity of local boards of health to assess and assure the health of communities, and inform local, state, and national policies that impact community health. The Massachusetts consortium also wanted to develop and institutionalize new, long-term, collaborative, and sustainable linkages among schools of public health and medicine, boards of health, and community-based organizations. Their belief was that community health could be improved by increasing partners' skills, and breaking the isolation of organizations so they could begin to work in full collaboration with people in communities.

The **Michigan** consortium planned to determine how academic and practice partners could catalyze health improvements in two targeted urban communities. Three teams were to be formed: one for the Genesee County-Flint community, one for a large neighborhood in northwest Detroit, and one for the academic community. The university was to be a member of the community teams, and each community a member of the academic team. The School of Public Health would become a coordinating bridge between the two urban teams. Two levels of program activities were planned. At

one level, each community would carry out a set of activities to promote interaction among team members, efforts that were likely to improve social and preventive health services through innovative programs and approaches with community residents. With the campus community, community-based approaches to public health problems were to be incorporated into the curriculum, student field-learning experiences, and research. All three teams would implement programs to expand career opportunities in health for economically disadvantaged youth.

The **North Carolina** consortium proposed to improve the health of minority and high-risk populations in selected communities by establishing collaborative structures and processes that responded to, empowered, and facilitated communities in defining and solving their own problems. All county coalitions would have some commonalities. Each planned to use lay health advisers/advocates as part of their action plan, and all were to conduct focus group discussions to identify specific commonalities and community needs. All agreed to participate fully with student rotations, and all identified the need for training both community leaders and agency personnel.

Within the consortium, specific coalitions pursued local objectives. The Wake County Coalition, with its major base in Raleigh, wanted to work with its urban community through Strengthening the Black Family, Inc., to bring programs, services, and information about health care, leadership development, economic development, and organizational support services closer to the people. The Orange County Coalition proposed to improve the health of minority groups in the Efland-Cheeks communities, helping residents assess and address their own special health problems. A Community Voices leadership program was to be used in conjunction with Chatham County, adapted from the local Cooperative Extension Service. The Chatham County Coalition hoped to improve the overall health and well-being of the residents of the Jordan Grove and Lincoln Heights communities. Efforts were to focus primarily around issues of obtaining safe water, adequate sewage disposal, and improved housing conditions. The Lee County Coalition hoped to foster community involvement in two public housing developments, enhance the leadership skills of the resident councils, and improve the health status of housing residents.

The **Washington** consortium proposal was designed as a collaborative model of education, practice, and research to improve the health of the target populations in inner Seattle and in the Lummi Indian Reservation near the Canadian border. Institutional change at the University of Washington was to facilitate the preparation of public and allied health professionals, and changes at the two health departments were to incorporate community issues into public health action and practice. The number, quality, and relevance of educational and professional development opportunities were to increase. A collaborative, policy-driven agenda was planned to emphasize community capacity building, inform policy options within the context of community issues, recruit and assist with upward mobility of youth of color, and embrace the racial, cultural, and economic differences of the partners. The initiative was to be grounded in shared risks, responsibilities, and rewards.

## Implementation, Year 1

The first year of the CBPH Initiative required attention to organizational issues. Staff and volunteers had to be recruited and trained, community and consortium meetings organized, and literally hundreds of new people incorporated into project activities. The CBPH approach had to be explained to new participants since the consortia were not typical partnerships and most partners had not worked together before. Consortia also needed to address mistrust between some partners, often based on valid historic reasons.

This early implementation period turned out to be crucial to setting the initiative's process in place. The expectation that the leaders who had been so immersed in the Leadership and Model Development year activities would guide the process turned out to be inaccurate. Having invested time in travel and planning, many of those who had become enthusiastic about the potential for community and public health change had to return to family and work responsibilities, leaving newly hired staff to provide the leadership for implementation. As a result, the replication process was imperfect in a number of sites. In retrospect it would have been better if leadership year activities had been repeated for new staff and partners. Over the next four years, as new people joined the project, all needed formal orientation to community-based concepts and approaches.

During the first year, a great deal of effort was expended organizing the local and national evaluation teams. This process was particularly difficult in some sites where community people suspected evaluators would become "intelligence agents" snooping into their affairs. And since so much information had to flow from the local sites to the cluster evaluation team, solid lines of communication between local and national evaluators was essential. To facilitate this exchange, common definitions of evaluation indicators and questions had to be agreed on, and the process of gathering and assimilating data had to be similar across sites.

Cluster evaluation team members and Kellogg Foundation staff independently made site visits to each of the projects during Year 1 and annually thereafter. The purpose of the visits was not to judge progress on a scale of prior expectations, but to better understand what was happening at the local level and get to know the people who were leading the effort. After a few months all project directors and local evaluators had been chosen, and it was possible to have monthly conference calls with each group to stay abreast of activities. Calls and site visits also were designed to inculcate the vision and purposes of CBPH to those who had not been involved during the initial year of Leadership and Model Development. A monthly newsletter, *CBPH News*, was produced and disseminated by the Foundation to facilitate communication and create a sense of national momentum. Local activities were featured in each edition.

Additional initiative-wide support was envisioned to advance CBPH goals. Specific support activities included: (1) networking, (2) publicity and promotion, (3) technical assistance, (4) evaluation, (5) leadership training, and (6) informing policymakers. But over time grantees indicated it would be better if publicity, technical assistance, leadership preparation, and policy support came directly from the local projects. Related issues are discussed at greater length in the following chapters.

The first administrative network meeting was held in Tucson, Arizona, in January 1993, and three representatives from each consortium attended. In later years this became the project directors/coordinators meeting, but some of the consortia still did not have a permanent staff leader at the time of the Tucson meeting. Planned as a working meeting, discussions were focused on governance and procedural issues. Attendees also were able to connect with other Kellogg Foundation grantees at the Community Partnerships with Health Professions Education Initiative meeting being held in Tucson at the time.

In April 1993, consortium-level evaluators met in Minneapolis to finalize agreement on the interplay between local and cluster evaluations. Evaluation questions and anticipated outcomes were negotiated as well

8

as the methods for gathering information (site visits, mailed surveys, videotaping) and indicator documentation. Guiding questions were: (1) What kinds of models were developed by CBPH consortia? (2) To what extent did participation affect the communities' capacity to solve public health problems? (3) To what extent did participation affect the capacity of member organizations to carry out their CBPH missions? (4) To what extent did participation affect the capacity of consortia members to influence policy? (5) For individuals and organizations involved, did the benefits of participation in CBPH outweigh the costs?

Seventy CBPH participants from all seven states attended the First Annual CBPH Network Meeting in Ann Arbor, Michigan, in June. Tours were made to Detroit's Agape House neighborhood and to the McCree North area of Flint to learn how people "on the ground" were responding to the challenges of the CBPH project. In Detroit, site visitors saw community health and social programs that were sponsored by an influential church and its urban partners. The group's village health worker training program and the health careers program for neighborhood youth attracted particular interest. In Flint, visitors saw a county health department that had moved aggressively to build bridges with neighborhood groups and collaborate as an equal in addressing community priorities. The visibility and prestige of the health agency had soared as a result, and its budget and programmatic efforts had moved ahead dramatically because of the support of elected officials.

The consensus from discussions at the meeting was that things were finally getting underway after a longer-than-expected startup period. Nearly 80 percent of the efforts during Year 1 had been directed to the community partners, preparing them for genuine collaboration with the public health professionals. Work had been initiated at the university level, particularly field work assignments for students. But relatively little activity was evident among most health agency partners. It was at this meeting that a decision was made about technical assistance for the individual consortia. Outside "experts" would not be routinely used, and the projects would rely on lessons learned from their peers in the CBPH Initiative. This led to exchange visits between consortium teams as a way of shared learning and growth, a powerful concept that was to become one of the backbones of the initiative over the coming months.

# Implementation, Year 2

In October 1993, public health agency representatives from six of the seven CBPH consortia met for a day-long discussion in Battle Creek, Michigan. The purpose was to identify opportunities and obstacles to change in local public health agencies, and to explore feasible strategies to achieving desired changes. The discussion was frank, animated, and invigorating. Most surprising was the relative unanimity within the group, given their disparate settings and responsibilities. Some of the agencies accepted the challenge to become mission-driven, choosing to improve outcomes by building community coalitions rather than simply adding new services. The group outlined a number of factors necessary to achieve the CBPH vision, some internal to agencies and others linked to relationships with community or academic partners. Factors that seemed most relevant to change were: (1) improving the skills of board members, managers, staff, and community; (2) addressing administrative and governance issues; (3) consolidating the funding streams; (4) growing diversity among staff to reflect the community; (5) creating managed care options in those agencies that have primary care responsibilities; (6) establishing a process to maintain agency focus; (7) building capacity to perform the core public health functions; (8) reviewing service utilization behaviors and practices; (9) learning to deal with highly mobile communities; (10) developing bridges to existing community assets; and (11) changing the perception of what a public health agency is and does.

That same month CBPH public health school deans gathered at the American Public Health Association meeting in San Francisco under the auspices of the Association of Schools of Public Health. Three items emerged from the discussion that merited action:

1. Deans needed ongoing communication and wanted to be included in the network activities;

2. Deans felt the university community largely misunderstood the CBPH Initiative (many felt that more community services were being requested of the university, when actually it was an opportunity to explore a new dimension of scholarship within the realm of community health); and

3. The sustainability of the projects needed more work, with a better understanding of how the community-academic partnerships could be institutionalized.

In December 1993 CBPH evaluators met again in Minneapolis, exploring the interface between project and cluster evaluation and clarifying roles. Peer support for building skills in data gathering and analysis was provided, and plans were made for videotape documentaries as a supplement to other forms of evaluation. A follow-up meeting in Battle Creek in May 1994 explored issues such as evaluation feedback loops and how to measure collaboration.

The project directors/coordinators also met in December 1993, convening in Oakland to share stories about their progress and talk about plans for the second operational year. For a full day they discussed the CBPH vision and what would be needed to realize that vision for the individual communities, health agencies, and university partners. They concluded by rewriting the vision statement for their own purposes:

The Community-Based Public Health (CBPH) Initiative is intended to bring renaissance to the field by strengthening the study, practice, and teaching of public health through creation of a broad array of new partnerships with an informed and involved public. The CBPH vision is of a community-driven public health discipline that achieves its goals of improved health and well-being through enhanced citizen input and action. This approach is in contrast to more traditional public health approaches that seek improved health indices through more and more services or new protocols for professional disease control, but with little help in planning or implementation from the community people at greatest risk.

In February 1994, the Foundation announced a new community challenge grant to stimulate consortia to begin raising funds from other sources to support program activities. In this new effort, the Foundation agreed to match, dollar for dollar, any amount raised up to $20,000 per community.

The Second Annual CBPH Network Meeting was held in Baltimore in June 1994, with more than 250 attendees. Michael McGinnis, Assistant Surgeon General and Director of the Office of Disease Prevention and Health Promotion, made three points as the keynote speaker: (1) the country needs to move from a focus on the Big 10 *diseases* to the Big 10 *causes* of illness; (2) we spend altogether too little on prevention; and (3) a community-based approach will be needed if the nation is to make a dent in these problems.

Two project updates provided useful benchmarks for charting progress. David Kears from Oakland shared his experiences in reorganizing the Alameda County Health Care Services Agency (home for the public health department), and Barbara Israel reported on the academic changes emanating from the CBPH project in the University of Michigan School of Public Health. Al Sommer, Dean of the Johns Hopkins University School of Hygiene and Public Health and official host for the meeting, reported on the discussions held by the public health deans earlier in the session. Site visits were made to several community churches in the East Baltimore area, hosted by Heart, Body, & Soul, Inc., and an evening celebration was held at the St. Francis Xavier Church, the oldest and largest African American Catholic congregation in the state. A number of small group workshops were offered to attendees. One of the new features was an International CBPH colloquium, with several representatives from South Africa and Brazil.

In July a publications task force was appointed to develop guidelines for attribution policies on future publications emanating from the CBPH projects.

The year ended with a growing understanding of the profound change that was being asked of CBPH partners. In almost every consortium the governance or decision-making structure had been pushed to its limits by very different partners, while being responsive to the challenge of collaboration. Some of the fledgling governance systems had become stronger and more self-confident over time, and their project activities had grown concomitantly. Other structures were dormant or had to be revised. In all instances, however, health advocacy in targeted communities had proceeded apace and had become the stabilizing centerpiece of CBPH work in Year 2.

## Implementation, Year 3

For most of Year 2 Kellogg Foundation program staff refined their own expectations for CBPH outcomes, particularly with reference to lessons learned from the evaluation. Communication and marketing plans were assembled to disseminate the information, and policy issues relevant to institutionalizing CBPH lessons were identified. Work related to evaluation, communication and dissemination, and policy was interconnected in the Initiative's Integrated Action Plan.

The Integrated Action Plan was presented at a joint meeting of project directors/coordinators and evaluators, held in Amherst, Massachusetts in October 1994. Although intended to assist CBPH partners in accomplishing initiative-wide objectives, the plan was not well received. Grantees perceived it as a top-down approach foreign to the philosophy of the entire CBPH Initiative. During a full day of heated discussion, consortia partners explained that they were still trying to resolve project-level decision systems and programs, and were not ready or willing to initiate work related to communication or informing policy discussions. The final outcome of the interchange was the proposed development of a three-tier approach in which:

1. Consorta would develop a project-level plan to communicate with stakeholders;

2. A National Policy Task Force would be appointed with input from each of the three partners (community, academe, and practice) from each state; and

3. The Foundation's work on an overall integrated action plan would continue and be updated and revised based on information from project-level plans and the Policy Task Force.

Beginning in Year 3, an increasing number of presentations on the CBPH Initiative were made. Panels at the American Public Health Association meeting reviewed various aspects of the program, including evaluation. Presentations were made to the senior center directors at the Centers for Disease Control and Prevention, Atlanta, and to senior staff at the Health Resources and Services Administration in Bethesda, Maryland. CBPH presentations were made at two workshops for the Agency for Health Care Policy and Research. CBPH speakers also were present at the Prevention '95 meeting and the executive and management committees of the Association of State and Territorial Officers (ASTHO) meeting in St. Louis. The Sun Valley Forum, an annual leadership conference held in Idaho, centered its 1995 meeting on new and developing schools of public health in America, and a major presentation was made on the CBPH Initiative and its impact on the future of public health education and research. Most of the individual consortia also made presentations to local groups.

In March 1995 a special meeting of the project directors/coordinators was held in Chicago to review progress in developing project-level communication plans. One of the needs expressed at the meeting was for a national clearinghouse to distribute such things as protocols, guidelines, course/curriculum information,

and other items that might be relevant to carrying out the CBPH mission. (It should be noted that the Center for the Advancement of Community Based Public Health was created in 1997 with this as one of its purposes.) During the second day of the meeting, attendees met with project directors from the parallel Community Partnerships with Health Professions Education Initiative. Conversation focused on future bridges between primary care and public health. Community was identified as a common partner that could facilitate connections between the two disciplines, and merged primary care and public health practices were seen as more responsive to community enhancement.

The CBPH National Policy Task Force also began work in the spring of 1995, convening its first formal meeting in May. For a report on the Task Force's efforts and lessons, please see Chapter VIII.

Two hundred twenty participants attended the Third Annual Network Meeting in Raleigh, North Carolina, in June 1995. The tone for the meeting was set by two keynote speakers: Reed V. Tuckson, president of Charles R. Drew University of Medicine and Science in Los Angeles, and Harry C. Boyte from the Center for Democracy and Citizenship at the University of Minnesota.

Tuckson talked about social stagnation that leads to hopelessness, indifference, inability to solve problems, and fear. His belief was that communities can work with institutions in programs of shared responsibility to address these problems. Boyte led with the observation that Americans have lost their touch for "government of and by the people," and talked about a sense of collective "public work" to lead the nation back to a more functional democracy. His ideas included: (1) citizens are the real producers, not government; (2) there is need for public space to carry out citizenship; (3) self-interest should not be interpreted as selfishness; (4) serving as a citizen is an art form that is learned over time, and ideas are the key, not techniques; (5) institutional changes are mandatory for the process to succeed; (6) public culture must be visible and seen as important; and (7) a commonwealth should be established within a larger vision so individuals can keep their eyes on the goal.

Small group sessions provided a venue for discussing the role of community health workers, community-based research, collaboration, academic policy changes, fund-raising, and other issues close to the work of CBPH partnerships. The International CBPH colloquium featured guests from Poland and Russia. Site visits were made to several of the rural project community sites in the North Carolina consortium.

Other miscellaneous activities during Year 3, carried out independently but in support of the initiative, included:

- Stakeholder focus groups, with a consultant hired to update strategies for promoting messages and lessons about the CBPH Initiative.

- Practice Partner mini-grants conceived to stimulate more public health agency projects (awards of up to $50,000 per CBPH agency).

- The Council on Linkages in Public Health was awarded a contract to begin the development of public health practice guidelines, in conjunction with the Centers for Disease Control and the U.S. Public Health Service.

- The Western Consortium for Public Health received a grant award to explore how public health leaders could carry out their mission in a managed care environment.

- The National Academy of Sciences received financial support for a Public Health Roundtable to update its 1988 study, *The Future of Public Health*.

- The American Public Health Association and the American Medical Association were aided in launching a national joint dialogue.

- The Hastings Center was awarded funds to examine the major ethical/moral and social arguments, and the cultural obstacles, in increasing the role of public health within the U.S. health care system.

- The Hospital Research and Education Trust, an arm of the American Hospital Association, was funded to conduct a national leadership action forum aimed at linking communities with the public and private sectors for purposes of health improvement.

## Implementation, Year 4

With the end of CBPH funding in sight, individual consortia began the fourth project year with a serious effort at local fund-raising and an examination of the aspects of project work that should be sustained. Throughout the year, much of the work took place in special committees, including the National Policy Task Force and the Communications Task Force. Efforts continued at the project level to build and focus the capacity of the partnerships on meaningful endeavors aimed at producing healthier communities. Yet there was a growing apprehension that the programs engendered through CBPH partnerships might be phased

back or phased out if resources could not be identified to continue the work.

The Fourth Annual Network Meeting, held in Washington, D.C., in June 1996, reflected the creativity and energy of Year 4. The meeting's 200 delegates focused on policy issues at the local, state, and national levels, and the communication and marketing required to spur positive system changes. The most important agenda item was review and approval of the National Policy Task Force recommendation that a new Center for the Advancement of Community Based Public Health be created, and vested with the power and resources to change the seven distinct but interconnected CBPH projects into a national movement. Task Force recommendations were adopted unanimously by the representatives, and the transformation process was officially underway.

The featured speaker for the celebratory dinner was Samuel Proctor, Professor Emeritus of Rutgers University and Duke Divinity School, and one of America's most famous preachers. He captured the spirit of true celebration, and the dinner ended with awards and spontaneous comments from the audience on ways the CBPH philosophy had influenced their thinking and changed lives.

The next day was filled with workshops on (1) transition management; (2) spirituality and health outcomes; (3) faith community and health ministries; (4) public opinion research findings; (5) a "Community Building" computer simulation offered by HealthCare Forum in San Francisco; and (6) the information superhighway and CBPH communities. The featured luncheon speaker was Antonia Novello, former U.S. Surgeon General and UNICEF Special Representative for Health and Nutrition. She talked about the special role of health professionals and well-informed community health workers in international development.

## Post-Implementation Phase

The work of community-based public health did not end with the conclusion of the CBPH Initiative. Most of the consortia were able to operate for several months and provide a transition for continuing the most vital parts of project work through volunteer efforts and funding from other sources.

Kellogg Foundation investment in the successor organization, the Center for the Advancement of Community Based Public Health, with the Group Health Cooperative of Puget Sound as fiscal agent, provided a solid beginning for the next phase. An invitational meeting held in Seattle in June 1997 for community representatives, policy task force members, and other key CBPH leaders initiated the work. The meeting marked two related events: the establishment of the new National Community-Based Organizations Network (NC-BON), and the formal beginning of the Center for the Advancement of Community Based Public Health (CA-CBPH).

The rationale for NC-BON was that while most public health professionals had their own organizations and societies, community organizations – the heart of the CBPH Initiative over the four-year period – had no equivalent structure. Initially NC-BON was operated as a subsidiary of the new CA-CBPH organization. CA-CBPH is now based in Durham, North Carolina, and is directed by a former community leader from the North Carolina CBPH consortium. CA-CBPH operates with a national Board of Directors comprised of experienced individuals from the seven-state CBPH consortia.

12

*Editors' Note: Chapter II describes a philosophy at the core of the Community-Based Public Health Initiative — the role of ordinary citizens in addressing complex societal problems. In contrast to the traditional emphasis on using technology and professional specialization to deal with challenges, Professor McKnight explains why those who have the most at stake in community issues need to be brought into the decision-making loop — and how their insights and contributions catalyze solutions to longstanding problems.*

| | |
|---|---|
| **Chapter II** | # Rationale for a Community Approach to Health Improvement |

*John L. McKnight*

We have clearly entered a new era in popular conceptions of health. Where once health was viewed as a *commodity* produced by medical systems, today there is a widespread recognition that health is also a *capacity* that can be maintained or enhanced by the ordinary citizen. Under the new era's banners of prevention and health promotion, corporate well-being programs appear and consciousness of health among Americans of all ages grows.

The new pro-health consciousness has created a hidden dilemma for health professions and professionals. That dilemma is most clearly manifested in the ever-growing professional use of the term "community." Under prevention and promotion rubrics, we hear of "community education," "community-based programs," "community participation," and so on. However, the meaning of "community" is not clear. At the very least, community usually means "not in a hospital, clinic or doctor's office." Community is the great "out thereness" beyond the doors of professional offices and facilities. It is the social space beyond the edges of our professionally run systems.

The dilemma we face is that while we have great professional skills in managing and working within our systems, our skills are much less developed once we leave the system's space and cross the frontier into "the community." Indeed, one is impressed by the immediate confusion and frustration experienced by many professionals when they attempt to work in community space, for it often seems very complex, dis-ordered, unstructured, and uncontrollable. And many health professionals begin to discover that their powerful tools and techniques seem weaker, less effective, and even inappropriate in the community.

It is because of this dilemma that some health professionals have begun to think more carefully about this social space called "the community." They have attempted to better understand how their profession can be more effective and which tools are needed for work in community space.

The most obvious finding of these professionals is best summarized by Mark Twain's maxim that, "If your only tool is a hammer, all problems look like nails." If your only tools are based upon medical models and systems, "the community" must be a nail if we are to be effective. However, with even the slightest reflection one can quickly recognize that the community is not a nail. It is, instead, a tool that is as distinctive and useful as the medical system tool.

In order to understand these distinctive tools called "health system" and "community" we need to look at the design, capacities, and appropriate use of each. Just as we can readily distinguish the different shape and use of a hammer and saw, it is possible to examine the distinctive shape and usefulness of a medical/health system and a community.

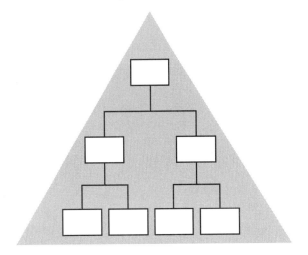

13

This article was previously published under the title of *Two Tools for Well-Being.*

Looking first at the tool we create called a system, its design or shape is best exemplified by the well-known organization chart that is a pyramid of boxes connected by lines of authority and responsibility. This pictograph of our medical, prevention, and health promotion systems should clarify the nature of the tool professionals use, a tool of which they are also a part.

This "system tool" is primarily designed to allow a few people to control many other people. It enables a manager or administrator to design and assure a standard output from the work of diverse professionals and workers. Therefore, it is clearly a tool designed to control and to produce standardized practices and outcomes. We can usually understand the nature of this system tool most clearly when we think about the production of an automobile. Here a pyramidal system is used to translate from the minds of a few designers and administrators to the hands of many technicians and workers a uniformly repetitive commodity called a Chevrolet. The auto company is a system designed to control in order to assure uniform quality in mass production. This is also the essential nature of the tool we call a medical or health system.

While systems are tools for creating control and uniform, repetitive quality, they also depend upon a third element of social organization: a consumer or a client. The frequent use of the words consumer and client is a product of modern system development and proliferation. Indeed, it has only been in the last 35 years that a previously unknown label was created by medical systems – the "health consumer." Our grandparents could not imagine such a being. They thought health was a condition, not a commodity. However, our new powerful systems have both needed and created a class of people called consumers and clients.

Therefore, we can recognize that the tool we use called a system is designed to control people in order to produce uniform goods and services of quality and to expand the number of people who act as consumers and clients.

What kind of tool is "the community?" It is obviously not a nail to be hammered by the health and medical systems. However, we must be somewhat arbitrary in our answer because there is no widely accepted definition of the design and shape of the "out thereness" often called community. Nonetheless, there is at least one very useful definition of the community that focuses upon a uniquely American social tool. This tool was first described and analyzed by a brilliant young Frenchman named Alexis de Tocqueville, who toured the United States in 1831.

In his monumental work titled *Democracy in America* (1966), Tocqueville observed that we had cre-

ated a new social tool in our neighborhoods. It was a self-generated local gathering of common people who assumed three powers: the power to decide what was a problem, to decide how to solve the problem, and the power to take action to carry out the solution. This powerful new tool he called an "association" and its members were called citizens.

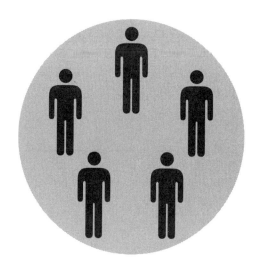

Tocqueville saw that our principal American tool for creating the new society was these self-appointed, self-defining assemblies of citizens. He recognized that they were, in their local aggregate, the new community of the New World – a universe of associated citizens. And through the mutually supportive associations, he saw the creation of citizen power that led to a powerful new form of *Democracy in America*.

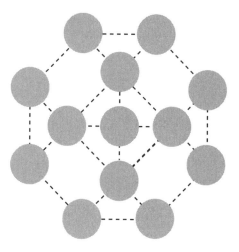

If we examine the nature of our current community of associations, we will see that they are tools with a special shape, design, and use that define a community's capacity.

First, associations are structures that depend upon the active consent of people. Unlike a system, the associational structure is not designed for the control of people. Systems ultimately depend upon people bending their uniqueness to a professional vision in exchange for money and security. Associations depend upon the consent of free individuals to join in equally expressing their creative and common visions.

Second, associations provide a context where care can be expressed. This contrasts with a system where standardized outcomes called services are the principle expression. Thus, at a gathering of an association of citizens, we see a social form that depends on consent and care. These elements in their unique combination by citizens create a social tool that is distinct from systems and with capacities different than those possessed by systems.

Third, associations require citizens rather than clients or consumers. Citizen is a political term. It describes the most powerful person in a democracy. An association is a tool to magnify the power of citizens. This contrasts with system tools that create and magnify clients. The Greek root of the word client is "one who is controlled." This is, of course, the opposite of a citizen who is one who holds power.

A community of associations, then, is a social tool that is designed to operate through consent, combining the creative uniqueness of the participants into a more powerful form of expression. Put simply, the unique American community is an assembly of associations that is the vital center of our democracy, our creativity, and our capacity to solve everyday problems.

What has this associational community to do with health? We can best understand if we review the epidemiology of health in a modern society.

I think it is generally agreed that there are five determinants of health:

- Individual behavior
- Social relations
- Physical environment
- Economic status
- Access to therapy

The first four are impervious to medicine. But they can be treated by citizens and their associations. Unfortunately, this vital health tool has been weakened since Tocqueville's observations of our social structures in 1831. Today, the power of American associations in community is less visible and less respected. The reason for the apparent decline of our community of associations is not very obvious to most of us, even though it has been clearly defined by such brilliant social analysts as Ivan Illich (1976), Jacques Ellul (1965), and Robert Bellah (1985). Their work demonstrates that the weakening of the tools of community is the direct result of the increasing power of the tools of systems. Indeed, they suggest a paradox – a zero-sum game. Their finding is that as the power of system tools grows, the power of community tools declines. As control magnifies, consent fades. As standardization is implemented, creativity disappears. As consumers and clients multiply, citizens lose power.

The implications of this analysis are profound. For if our health tool is a system, we can only achieve a particular and limited set of goals. We cannot perform the necessary functions and achieve the goals of the tools of community. And yet, it is critical to health promotion and prevention that most of the work be done in and *by* communities.

Some modern health professionals, recognizing this necessity, have begun to design complex programs said to "interface with," "involve" or "use" the community. As noble as their intentions may be, they fail to recognize the historical evidence demonstrating that as systems grow in capacity, influence, and power, communities and their associations lose capacity, influence, and power (Polanyi, 1944). As systems "outreach," communities contract. As systems invade, associations retreat.

As we enter the era that seeks healthy communities, we are faced with four hard realities. First, systems and communities are different tools designed to do different work. Second, systems can never replace the work of communities. Third, system growth and outreach can diminish and erode the power of the community's tools. Fourth, when systems' growth erodes community associations, then the system itself becomes a major cause of community weakness and disempowerment contributing to the creation of a local environment for ill-health, un-wellness and dis-ease. Put simply, powerful, pervasive health systems can create unhealthy communities by replacing consent with control and active citizens with compliant clients.

In the face of these hard realities, there are no easy tricks or technical gimmicks that health professionals can use to overcome either the limits or the potential counterproductivity of health system tools. There are, however, some hopeful experiments and initiatives in which health professionals and their powers have enhanced the strength of communities and their associations. Our analysis of these cooperative initiatives suggest that they reflect at least four values.

First, the professionals have a deep respect for the wisdom of citizens in association. These professionals do not speak of training or paying citizens or associations to do the system's work. Rather, they seem to recognize that they are fellow citizens with one symbolic vote to use in association with their fellow citizens. While they are not a part of the community, they walk with the community on its journey. They are neither making the path nor leading the group.

Second, community-building professionals often have useful health information for local folks. They share that information in understandable forms. For example, they prepare a map that shows where neighborhood auto accidents occurred last year. They ask local citizens in their associations why the accidents occurred and what the local citizens association can do about the problem. They are not the source of analysis or solutions. They are the source of information that is not easily known by local citizens. They provide information that mobilizes the power of local citizen associations to develop and implement solutions (McKnight, 1978).

Third, they use their capacities, skills, contacts, and resources to strengthen the power of local associations. They are listening for opportunities to enhance local leadership, strengthen local associations, and magnify community commitments. They are not trying to gain space, influence, credit, or resources for their system. Instead, they are asking how the system's resources might enhance the problem-solving capacities of local groups.

Finally, the new community-building health professionals are escaping the ideology of the medical model. For all its utility, the medical model always carries with it a hidden negative assumption. That assumption is that what is important about a person is their injury, their disease, their deficiency, their problem, their need, their empty half. This deficiency perspective usually leads to the same kind of focus in communities. The result is the typical map of a neighborhood that is created from a "needs survey."

## Neighborhood Needs Map

16

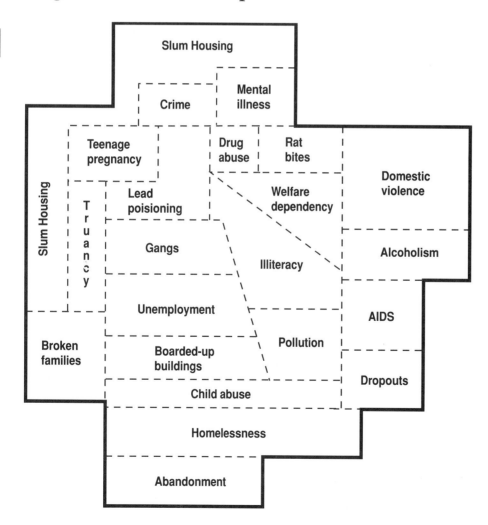

The part of a person that is able, gifted, skilled, capable and full is not the focus of the medical model. And yet, communities are built upon the capacities of people – not their deficiencies. Therefore, the essential map of a healthful community identifies the local assets rather than needs.

Communities are built by one-legged carpenters. Medical systems are built on the missing leg. It is for this reason that community health professionals inevitably find that they must invert the medical model and focus on capacities rather than needs and deficiencies (Kretzmann and McKnight, 1993). They must understand the map of community capacity.

Initiatives that enhance healthy associative communities are necessarily built upon the identification and expression of the gifts, skills, capacities, and associations of citizens. And so it is that community-building professionals are not interested in how many girls are parents too soon. Rather, they are interested in what these same girls can contribute to the community. How are they connected to local associations to express their gifts? What existing groups will give them a new source of power and identity? What can I, and the resources of my system, do to join the effort to answer these questions without overwhelming or co-opting local citizen efforts?

## Neighborhood Assets Map

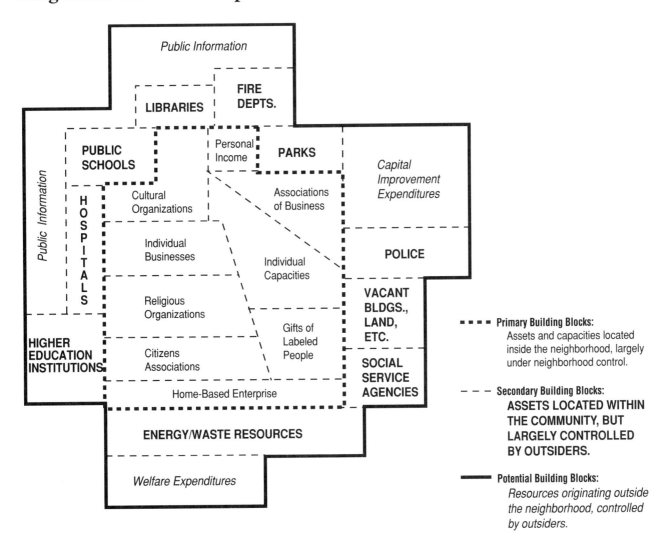

In order to build a healthful society, we need two tools. One is a system. The other is a community. Neither can substitute for the other, but systems can displace communities or enhance them. To enhance community health, we need a new breed of modest health professionals. They will be people with a deep respect for the integrity and wisdom of citizens and their associations. They will understand the kinds of information that will enable citizens to design and solve problems. They will direct some system resources to enhancing associational powers. And above all, they will focus upon magnifying the gifts, capacities, and assets of local citizens and their associations.

Health is not an input. Health is not a commodity. Health cannot be consumed.

Health is a condition. Health is a byproduct of strong communities. Health is the unintended side effect of citizens acting powerfully in association. Without that citizen power in associative relationships, we will be reduced to a nation of clients – impotent consumers feeling the unhealthful dis-ease from the manipulation of our lives as they are managed and controlled by hierarchical systems.

Alexis de Tocqueville had it right in 1831. He saw a vital, creative, vigorous, lively, inventive, healthful people. He understood that was because they were neither clients nor consumers. Instead, they were citizens and that fact was the source of their health and their healthful communities.

Tocqueville thought he was a reporter. But he was also a prophet who understood that the basic source of health is powerful citizens and vigorous associations. The name he gave to that health-giving condition was democracy.

## References

Bellah RN, Madsen R, Sullivan WM, Swidler A, Tipton SM. *Habits of the Heart: Individualism and Commitment in American Life.* Berkeley, CA: University of California Press; 1985.

Ellul J. *The Technological Society.* New York: Knopf Publishers; 1965.

Illich I. *Medical Nemesis: The Expropriation of Health.* New York: Pantheon Books; 1976.

Kretzmann J, McKnight J. *Building Communities From the Inside Out: A Path Toward Finding and Mobilizing a Community's Assets.* Evanston, IL: Center for Urban Affairs and Policy Research Report, Northwestern University; 1993.

McKnight J. Politicizing health care. *Social Policy.* 1978; 9:36-9.

Polanyi K. *The Great Transformation.* New York: Farrar and Rinehart Publishing; 1944.

deTocqueville A. *Democracy in America.* New York: Harper and Row; 1966.

*Editors' Note: In the following chapter, three eminent authorities on public health and the American health care system provide an overview of the profession at the outset of a new century. Drs. Paxman, Lee, and Satcher review the history and present condition of public health and provide insight into the future of the profession in light of current political, social, scientific, and economic trends, and within the context of the health care marketplace.*

# Chapter III | Public Health Status at the Beginning of the Twenty-First Century

*Dalton G. Paxman, Philip R. Lee, and David Satcher*

## Introduction

The challenges facing public health at the dawn of the twenty-first century are much as they were more than a decade ago when the Institute of Medicine (IOM) issued its report, *The Future of Public Health* (1988). These challenges, and some of the major efforts that have been made to address them at the national, state, and local levels, have been reviewed in a series of reports over the last decade. These include a United States Public Health Service (PHS) report, *For a Healthy Nation: Returns on Investment in Public Health* (1995), articles by Breslow (1990), Lee and Paxman (1997), Baker et al. (1994), Lasker (1997), and the IOM report, *Healthy Communities: New Partnerships for the Future of Public Health* (1996).

The IOM's Committee on the Future of Public Health defined public health in the following way:

> *Public health is what we, as a society, do collectively to assure the conditions in which people can be healthy. This requires that continuing and emerging threats to the health of the public be successfully countered. These threats include immediate crises, such as the AIDS epidemic; enduring problems, such as injuries and chronic illness; and impending crises foreshadowed by such developments as the toxic byproducts of a modern economy* (1988).

We would reemphasize the pertinence of several of the problems that were identified in the report, including tobacco use, alcohol and illicit drug abuse, injuries (intentional and unintentional), asthma, and teenage pregnancy. Today the public health and medical care

*Public health is what we, as a society, do collectively to assure the conditions in which people can be healthy.*

response to terrorism, whether through nuclear, chemical, biological, or conventional weapons, must be added as a public health responsibility. Greater emphasis should also be given now to prevention, particularly in such areas as physical activity, nutrition, food safety, and early childhood development.

Historically, in addition to the traditional focus of public health agencies on clean water and safe food supplies, the profession has enjoyed some notable successes. The PHS report identified these as including the virtual elimination of polio, declines in dental decay due to fluoridated community water supplies, and reductions in childhood blood lead levels through the elimination, by regulation, of lead in gasoline. These are problems that demand continued attention and the unique competence of public health practitioners.

Fogel stressed the importance of nutrition in improving the public's health in his 1993 Nobel Prize lecture for economic sciences (1994). He traced the impact of economic development on the nutritional/health status of the populations in the United Kingdom, France, and the United States since 1700. He estimated that improvements in nutrition had increased productivity per capita by 30 percent between 1790 and 1980. No other single factor was so important. He also noted the long-term health impacts of social infrastructure investments (e.g., sewage systems, safe water supplies) that were made after the turn of the century.

In this chapter, we will consider public health and its challenges within the context of social, political, economic, scientific, and technological changes that are affecting the United States, and indeed the rest of the world, in the transition from an industrial age to an information age in the 21st century. We also will examine the progress that has been made in the past decade in addressing major threats to health, in creating a public health infrastructure for the future, in addressing the challenge of managed care, in fostering public-private partnerships, particularly at the community level, and in assuring accountability. Finally, we will emphasize those areas where public health solutions come from community-based partnerships.

## Political, Social, and Economic Forces Shaping Public Health

The United States is an aging and increasingly diverse society that is changing because of the growing number of elderly and the rapid rise in immigration from Asia, Mexico, and the Caribbean in the past 20 years. Politically, the antipathy to these new immigrants on the part of largely second and third generation European immigrants is resulting in punitive policies that deny a variety of social welfare, medical care, and education benefits to immigrants, both legal and illegal.

In this environment, health policy at the federal level is viewed within a broad political context, as analyzed by Brinkley, Polsby, and Sullivan in *New Federalist Papers* (1997). In his preface to this brilliant series of essays dealing with fundamental political issues, Richard C. Leone notes:

> The assault on government threatens the fundamentals of the American system; it has taken shape in a host of legislative initiatives and hundreds of proposed amendments to the Constitution. What is perhaps most remarkable is the fact that so many amendments are being given serious consideration in Congress (p. vii).

The willingness of the second-term Clinton White House and the Republican-controlled Congress to compromise, moving away from the gridlock that characterized the 1994-1996 period, led to agreements on welfare reform, minimum wage, and the balanced budget agreement. These compromises will shape the context within which public health policies will be decided at the outset of this new century. Perhaps the most important is the balanced budget agreement reached in 1997.

Under that agreement, reductions were mandated in anticipated Medicare expenditure increases before 2002, loosened somewhat by Congress in November 1999. Seventeen billion dollars was added to expand health insurance for children, through either Medicaid or private insurance, and limits were placed on domestic discretionary spending.

The budget agreement and a booming economy led to one of the last substantial policy debates between the Clinton Administration and Congress, namely how to spend the forecasted budget surplus. At the turn of this century, budget analysts predict nearly $1 trillion in estimated budget surpluses over 10 years. The surpluses have led to verbal sparring over competing priorities for the allocation of these resources. Congressional leadership called for massive tax cuts to return money to taxpayers, while the White House called for smaller tax cuts and the remaining surplus targeted at Medicare, Social Security, and other social programs. As of this writing no agreements have been reached, although public opinion seems to favor paying down the national debt over either large tax cuts or new social spending.

In light of the competition over spending priorities, the results of a survey sponsored by the Pew Charitable Trust seem telling. Two-thirds of respondents believe that more should be done to protect the public's health. An overwhelming number agreed that the U.S. should spend more for public health than other priorities, including tax cuts, fighting crime, building roads, and the missile defense system (Pew Commission Website, www.pewenvirohealth.jhsph.edu).

Efforts to curb tobacco use will continue as a major public health priority in the twenty-first century. The Clinton Administration sought to regulate cigarettes by controlling nicotine through both the FDA's drug and device authorities. A decision by the U.S. Court of Appeals to invalidate the regulation of tobacco products by the FDA is being appealed to the Supreme Court. An *amicus curiae* brief submitted by the American Cancer Society urges a reversal of the appellate decision and makes an excellent case in support of the FDA's regulatory authority over tobacco products (1999).

With FDA's appeal awaiting a Supreme Court decision, most of the anti-tobacco efforts are directed at the multi-state lawsuit against the tobacco companies, which seeks to recover the costs to the state Medicaid programs from tobacco-related illnesses. The lawsuit forced the tobacco industry to agree to a settlement with state attorneys general. In addition to the billions of dollars to settle class action lawsuits, the settlement provides for a cigarette tax that will be used to fund smoking prevention and cessation programs and other public health education activities. Some states have allocated significant portions of the settlement for anti-tobacco programs; unfortunately, a number of states have decided not to apply their settlement funds to this end.

Economically, a host of factors affect the nation's future prospects for public health. During the latter half of the 1990s the country was doing very well compared to other industrialized nations, based on a number of economic indicators. These included a low rate of unemployment, a low level of inflation, millions of new jobs annually, a booming stock market, and strong corporate profits. How long this period of sustained growth will last is not clear. Certainly, the financial troubles in Asia, some Latin American countries, and Russia may have an impact on the U.S. economy over time.

There are other reasons for concern: while incomes of the top 10 percent of U.S. citizens have risen dramatically in the past decade, lower wage workers have seen a decline in income relative to rising costs, particularly before passage of the minimum wage increase in 1996. The gap in income between the rich and poor has widened, so that the U.S. now has the largest income gap of any of the industrialized nations – with negative health implications (Kreiger, Williams, and Moss, 1997). There also are some positives to be found in the current high level of employment and the growth in federal, state, and local tax revenues. In some states and in some local communities, additional resources are being directed to selected public health programs and agencies.

The global economy became a fact of life at the end of the 20th century, with implications for public health. The underlying premise of the tobacco settlement was that the export market for tobacco products to the Third World would eventually finance the health care costs of American smokers. While the United States *is* exporting more products, including airplanes, computers, and airmail services, it also is importing more fresh fruits and vegetables (especially from Mexico and Central America), beef (from Central and South America), seafood (from Asia), and other food products. All these present an increasing challenge to the FDA and state public health agencies to ensure the safety of the food supply.

The 1996 cyclospora outbreak related to Guatemalan raspberries and the 1997 hepatitis A outbreak related to Mexican strawberries illustrate the problem. It would now appear that the number of cases of foodborne illness is much greater than earlier believed. In the most complete estimate to date, the Centers for Disease Contol (CDC) determined that foodborne diseases may cause an estimated 325,000 serious illnesses in the United States each year that result in hospitalization, plus 76 million cases of gastrointestinal illnesses, and 5,000 deaths.

Environmental health concerns, such as global climate change and ozone depletion, also have significant implications for all countries.

## The Health Care Marketplace and the Advance of Science

The concept of health care as a market good – a commodity to be bought and sold – has come to prevail over the view of health care as a public good, an essential service performed for the benefit of the entire community (Lee, Benjamin, and Weber, 1997). Large employers, driven by a desire to reduce medical care costs, turned to managed care approaches during the 1990s, restricting employee benefits and physician choice, and increasing cost sharing by employees. Health coverage changes related to managed care (capitated payments, limited consumer choice, and a slowing of cost increases) have been accompanied by an increase in the number of uninsured by one million per year – 15 percent of the U.S. population in 1996. Dissatisfaction with HMO management of patient care resulted in both political parties attempting to establish a baseline of health care standards, which President Clinton termed a "Patient's Bill of Rights." Annas delineated issues surrounding patient's rights (1999). Disagreements within the Congress prevented the passage of a health care bill in 1999.

Science and technology remain of critical importance in health care. Many new technologies, such as vaccines and antibiotics, have had substantial benefits both to individuals and to the health of the population in the past 50 years, and many more will be forthcoming. Despite the advances, the emergence of newly identified infectious agents, such as E. *coli* 0157:H7, antibiotic-resistant microbes, and pesticide-resistant insects suggest that we cannot ignore public health threats we assumed were conquered in the past. Medical technology also continues to drive health care costs.

The future of public health will be influenced by: (1) the rapid advances in genetics stimulated by the Human Genome Project; (2) the growing importance of psychosocial factors affecting the health status of the population; (3) the rapid development of information systems technology; (4) developments in vaccine research and other biotechnologies; and (5) advances in nutrition.

## New Demands on Public Health

Throughout the twentieth century, with the exception of the 1918-1919 influenza epidemic, the mortality rate declined and life expectancy at birth increased. Breslow, in his *Annual Review of Public Health* (1990), described the dramatic improvements in health that accompanied the sanitary revolution and the application of the germ theory to public health in the late

21

nineteenth and the twentieth century (e.g., pasteurization of milk, chlorination of water supplies, vaccines, and antibiotics). These achievements also have been reviewed by Lee (1995), Duffy (1990), Fee (1991), and Fogel (1994).

In the United States, life expectancy increased from about 40 years in 1850 to 68 years in 1950 (Fogel, 1994). In the 1960s and 1970s, progress in longevity slowed as the chronic diseases (e.g., heart disease, cancer, and stroke) played an increasingly important role in the health of the population. What followed was the "second public health revolution" (Breslow, 1990; Fee, 1991), which reoriented public health toward a greater emphasis on chronic disease prevention. Attention shifted to identifying the causal factors of the major chronic diseases and how to intervene in an effective way. Collaboration between clinicians and public health practitioners resulted in a dramatic decline in mortality from heart disease and stroke. Public health's major contributions were risk assessment, population screening (hypertension), design and evaluation of clinical trials (tobacco control), the development of better vital and health statistics (NHANES, behavioral risk factor survey), and the development of improved performance measures.

The Centers for Disease Control estimate that public health has added 25 years to the life expectancy of people in the United States in this century. Despite this, the public remains largely unaware of the importance of public health. To overcome this lack of awareness, the CDC created the "Ten Greatest Public Health Achievements in the 20th Century" and ran a series of articles on these in the *Morbidity and Mortality Weekly Report* throughout 1999 (www.cdc.gov/epo/mmwr/preview/mmwrhtml/00056796.htm). The list includes immunizations, motor vehicle safety, workplace safety, control of infectious diseases, declines in deaths from heart disease and stroke, safer and healthier foods, healthier mothers and babies, family planning, fluoridation of drinking water, and tobacco as a health hazard.

At the end of the twentieth century chronic diseases – particularly cardiovascular disease, cancer, diabetes, and alcoholism – represent the greatest killers. Many other chronic diseases may be disabling (osteoarthritis, osteoporosis, cataracts) but rarely cause death. Injuries, both unintentional and intentional

*At the end of the twentieth century chronic diseases – particularly cardiovascular disease, cancer, diabetes, and alcoholism – represent the greatest killers.*

(child abuse, family violence), are also major public health problems.

Emerging health problems present another challenge to the nation's public health system (Institute of Medicine, 1988). Asthma, especially in children, has risen despite steadily improving air quality in our cities. Outbreaks of new infectious diseases such as HIV/AIDS, the Hanta virus in the Southwest, E. *coli* 0157:H7 in hamburgers, the Ebola virus in Zaire, and familiar diseases that have become resistant to therapeutic drugs (tuberculosis) illustrate the state of readiness public health agencies must maintain.

The growing number of uninsured places an additional burden on local health departments, often community providers of medical care in addition to their public health functions. As millions more people have lost private health insurance in the 1990s, public health and hospital officials at the local level increasingly have been left with the responsibility of providing medical care to the uninsured.

# The Public Health System

The *Future of Public Health* report (Institute of Medicine, 1988) created a conceptual framework for the three core functions of public health (assessment, assurance, policy development) and issued a wake-up call to public health leaders throughout the country. Since then, the U.S. Public Health Service, working with state and local health officials, has taken the lead in assessing the performance of public health agencies to carry out their societal missions. The goal of these efforts is to improve the performance of the public health system by continuing to examine and define not only core public health functions, but also the organizational framework and public health expenditures. This next section analyzes the core functions of public health and of the public health system.

# Core Functions of Public Health

The Essential Public Health Services work group has identified 10 public health services that describe public health's core assessment, policy, and assurance functions in more detail.

22

## Ten Essential Public Health Services

- Monitor health status to identify community health problems;

- Diagnose and investigate health problems and health hazards in the community;

- Inform, educate, and empower people about health issues;

- Mobilize community partnerships to identify and solve health problems;

- Develop policies and plans that support individual and community health efforts;

- Enforce laws and regulations that protect health and ensure safety;

- Link people to needed personal health services and assure the provision of health care when otherwise unavailable;

- Assure a competent public health and personal health care workforce;

- Evaluate effectiveness, accessibility, and quality of personal and population-based health services; and

- Research for new insights and innovative solutions to health problems.

*Source:* The Essential Public Health Services work group of the Core Public Health Functions Steering Committee/Office of the Assistant Secretary for Health, United States Department of Health and Human Services

These essential services support the specific design of public health agencies to:

- prevent epidemics and the spread of disease;

- protect against environmental hazards;

- prevent injuries;

- promote and encourage healthy behaviors;

- respond to disasters and assist communities in recovery; and

- assure the quality and accessibility of health services.

This list has been broadly used in the public health community to define workforce competencies, monitor expenditures, and in some cases reorganize health departments. Increasingly, given the public's confusion about the field, the list also is being used to explain public health functions and priorities to those outside the field.

While core public health functions describe the activity of public health broadly, they do not translate easily into population-based services actually provided in the community. Hence, the status of the public health infrastructure down to the local level has been difficult to assess. The Office of Public Health and Science at the Department of Health and Human Services (DHHS) funded studies to address this problem (Eilbert et al., 1997; Barry et al., 1998). The project used the 10 essential services as a method for quantifying public health expenditures at the state and local levels. While limited to nine states and three local sites, the pilot studies showed the feasibility of using the essential services to collect reliable public health expenditure data, which can contribute to a more rational approach to allocating scarce public health resources.

The proliferation of federal categorical grants in public health, particularly since the 1960s, has made it increasingly difficult for state and local health departments to set priorities and allocate resources according to the needs at the local level (Lee, Benjamin, and Weber, 1997). Categorical funding removes some of the flexibility necessary to allow local health officials to address the public health concerns of their own community.

## Public Health Practice

As Breslow noted, the 1988 IOM report gave a major stimulus to the reconstitution of public health (1990). While the need for reform is broadly recognized and while there is wide agreement on the basic premises, there is as yet little agreement on what constitutes public health at the local level, what the essential public health functions should be, or even what the current expenditures for public health ought to be. Work done in North Carolina, Illinois, and Washington (see below) lays the groundwork for a system of performance standards for local and state health agencies built around the 10 essential services. An excellent review by Turnock and Handler (1997) describes efforts to measure the extent and effectiveness of public health practice in the United States since 1900.

A study of local health departments by the National Association of County and City Health Officials (NACCHO), in cooperation with CDC, provides a snapshot of the current organization of public health agencies at the local level (U.S. Department of

23

Health and Human Services, 1995b). They surveyed 2,079 local health departments (72 percent of all local health departments) and found the following:

- 79 percent had a top agency executive.

- 73 percent are governed by a local board of health.

- 42 percent have fewer than 10 employees.

- Public health services provided included immunization (96 percent), tuberculosis control (86 percent), restaurant inspection and/or licensing (80 percent), well-child services (79 percent), water supply safety services (74 percent), and HIV/AIDS testing and counseling (68 percent).

The NACCHO/CDC survey results were similar to the findings of earlier studies by the School of Public Health, University of North Carolina (Brooks et al., 1976). The NACCHO/CDC study added a new service, HIV/AIDS counseling and testing, and an expanded role for local health departments in health care for the indigent.

The University of Illinois also developed its own assessment tool to measure the performance of local health departments. They found that the agencies surveyed performed about 50 percent of their work in association with 10 basic practices in the core functions of public health, including three assessment practices, three policy development practices, and four assurance practices (Institute of Medicine, 1996b). Performance was more extensive in larger health departments than in smaller departments. From the survey responses, they estimate that only about 20-30 percent of health departments (serving about 40 percent of the population of the United States) had an effective level of performance in terms of the *Healthy People 2000* objectives. "Effective" was defined as (1) performing 7 of 10 public health practices included in the list of core functions, or (2) performing at least two of the assessment practices, two of the policy development practices, and three of the assurance practices.

In Illinois, the performance of local health departments was reassessed in 1992 and 1994 using a set of 26 measures of public health practice (Turnock et al., 1995). They found that the percentage of practices performed rose from 55 percent to 85 percent between the two dates. The local health departments attribute this increase to the state requirement that they conduct regular assessments using NACCHO's APEXPH model (National Association of County and City Health Officials, 1991) or an Illinois version of this called I PLAN (Illinois Plan for Local Assessment of Needs).

To test the performance of local health departments, Rohrer et al. (1997) surveyed six states in 1993 and the Iowa health agency directors in 1995. In both surveys, performance of core public health practices averaged only about 50 percent. Performance was worst in the planning functions (assessment, investigation, planning, evaluation).

North Carolina also initiated a self-assessment program in 1992, following the directions of the state legislature. The state health department was asked to "implement a monitoring and evaluation program to measure local health department progress in applying health outcome standards and achieving health outcome objectives established by the commission for health services" (U.S. Department of Health and Human Services, 1995b). The North Carolina Task Force responded to the state legislature by developing a three-level accountability system:

**Level I.** Community Wellness Status indicators in eight broad categories: (1) maternal and child health; (2) child health; (3) heart disease and stroke; (4) cancer; (5) diabetes and other chronic diseases; (6) injury; (7) communicable diseases; and (8) adolescent health status.

**Level II.** Public health needs of the community and how needs are met by the health department and the community (indicators are population-based).

**Level III.** Program-specific assessments, generally to assure that local agencies are operating in compliance with state and federal regulations.

The task force concluded that the accountability process and the community diagnostic process are complementary. One represents an analysis undertaken at the state level concerning community health status and public health activities; the other represents a self-assessment at the community level of health status and service provision.

At the state level, agency reorganization has seemed to be in order through the 1900s, yet the reorganization has varied widely. In some states a reconstituted Department of Health has included public health and Medicaid. In others, public health has been created as a cabinet level department (Florida). In some, a variety of public health functions, including health statistics, alcohol and substance abuse, and mental health have been included within a single agency. Yet in other states these public health functions have remained sep-

24

arate. To date, little analysis has been reported on the impact of the state-level reorganization that has taken place in more than 20 states.

Like state governments, the federal government also has been reorganizing its public health structure. In an attempt to give public health higher priority and create a more efficient and decentralized management structure, a major "reinvention" of PHS was carried out in 1995. As a result, the Assistant Secretary for Health, DHHS, became the senior health and science advisor to the Secretary, instead of being the line manager of PHS. The Secretary, not the Assistant Secretary for Health (ASH), is the director of PHS, but the Surgeon General continues to report to the ASH. In President Clinton's second term, the same individual serves in both positions; this was also true for the Carter Administration.

What has been accomplished is a greater emphasis in DHHS and the White House on major public health issues – things like tobacco control, immunization, HIV/AIDS, women's health, physical activity, nutrition, newly emerging infectious diseases, environmental health, and performance objectives – and outcomes measurement in public health. These changes, while important, cannot substitute for the national health policy/management structures that will be needed to address the challenges of the twenty-first century.

Central to restructuring the public health system is the importance of public health information, its generation, dissemination, and communication. More needs to be known about the determinants of health, and key changes must be made to the entire system in order to achieve public health objectives, as well as to integrate our knowledge of these determinants. A framework for collecting and distributing public health information must be developed, not only to ensure access for all who will use it, but to protect against those who may misuse it. Finally, we must acknowledge the impact this information will have on the public and how to best foster communication with populations at risk.

## Expenditures for Public Health

The entire public health system is large and complex. While the private sector plays a dominant role in per-

*Central to restructuring the public health system is the importance of public health information, its generation, dissemination, and communication.*

sonal health care, the system receives large public subsidies in a variety of forms. Additionally, the role of federal and state governments is interwoven, and often overlapping, in both public health and health care financing. In 1996, total health expenditures exceeded one trillion dollars. The financing of personal health care dominated health expenditures at the federal and state levels, to the detriment of population-based interventions that have the goal of protecting and improving the public's health.

Currently, the national expenditure for population-based programs is estimated to be less than one percent of the aggregate amount spent for all health care in the United States. This estimate excludes environmental health programs, highway safety, occupational safety and health, and the Department of Agriculture's food program for women, infants, and children (WIC), along with its meat and poultry inspection programs. A 1996 study (Levit et al.) outlined the federal government's health expenditures. From a total of $1,035.1 billion, approximately 88 percent ($907.2 billion) was for personal health care; 5.9 percent ($60.9 billion) for program administration and the net cost of health insurance; 3 percent ($31.5 billion) for research and construction; and 3.4 percent ($35.5 billion) for government public health activities. In the last category, only $3.8 billion went to federal public health agencies and the remaining $27.6 billion to state and local agencies. In contrast, Medicare expenditures totaled $203.1 billion in 1996, and federal/state and local Medicaid expenditures were $147.7 billion. For these two personal health care programs alone, expenditures are about 10 times those for all public health agencies.

As was discussed earlier, due to the rapid changes in the finance and delivery of health care in the United States, the Public Health Foundation (PHF) developed an approach for measuring public health expenditures (Eilbert et al., 1997). Although the results were limited to pilot studies in nine states, certain trends were clearly identified. Of an estimated $8.8 billion in public health agencies, PHF found that 69 percent was spent on personal health services, while 31 percent was spent on population-based health services. At the same time, state and local health departments have become major providers of personal health services to medically indigent populations (Lee, Benjamin, and Weber, 1997).

25

Using this distribution of funds for personal and population-based health services for the 1996 expenditures for governmental health activities, population-based prevention shrinks to approximately one percent of national health expenditures.

PHF also demonstrated the feasibility and utility of using the essential services framework to determine local public health expenditures (Barry et al., 1998). However, there were problems of comparability and reliability. Despite their limitations, both the state and local expenditure studies provide a starting point for estimating public health expenditures and improving policy decisions in the future.

## Public Health Infrastructure

Strengthening the public health system for this new century will require focusing on three areas: research, workforce, and information systems.

### Research

Studies now underway seem likely to shape both public health and personal health care in the future. From the human genome project to studies on the effects of social class on health, research is rapidly transforming our understanding of the variety of factors (biological, behavioral, social, environmental) that converge to influence health. It is critical to apply this knowledge to health policy and clinical and public health practice.

Prevention research is the foundation for both clinical preventive services and population-based health intervention. The nation's substantial investments in research thus far have focused far more on biomedical approaches to prevention than on behavioral, socioeconomic, or environmental factors that contribute to health status. Evaluating the costs and effectiveness of personal and population-based services is also vastly underfunded. Future investments in research need to support a balance between highly focused and broad-range multidisciplinary research in areas that include basic biological sciences, clinical medicine, public health practice, the behavioral and social sciences, epidemiology, health systems and services, occupational health and safety, and environmental

health. The biological pathways that translate socioeconomic factors into immunological or endocrinological changes also need to be better understood. Nutrition, although critical to human health, is not adequately studied by the National Institutes of Health or the Department of Agriculture (USDA).

Continued public support is necessary to revise priorities toward increased emphasis on nutritional, environmental, behavioral, and social science research, as well as information systems research.

### Workforce

The health workforce is the backbone of both the personal health care and public health systems. While ample evidence has accumulated about workforce issues that must be addressed in medicine and the allied health professions (O'Neil, 1993; Rivo and Kindig, 1996; Rivo and Satcher, 1993), far less attention has been paid to the need for training in population-based health (U.S. Department of Health and Human Services, 1994 and 1997c). There are serious shortages in some public health specialty areas (e.g., epidemiology) and many individuals in the current workforce need further training to effectively assess health problems and implement population-based strategies for improving health. To build a workforce that supports the emerging managed care environment, schools for the health professions must work to address the needs of the system and the diversity of the population.

Health professionals also need to be trained to work effectively together, linking population-based public health and interdisciplinary clinical care. Current health care financing systems have created incentives for a physician workforce trained in high-cost, high-tech, episodic methods of care. The workforce also trains and utilizes too few nurse practitioners and other non-physician professionals. There are few medical school graduates who have had training in community-based and cost-effective approaches to practice. Thus, in its present configuration, the provider workforce and associated training programs are not well-matched to national needs.

The policies undergirding federal financing of graduate medical education (GME) and teaching hospitals are currently being evaluated. Federal outlays for

*The nation's substantial investments in research thus far have focused far more on biomedical approaches to prevention than on behavioral, socioeconomic, or environmental factors that contribute to health status.*

GME in 1997 were $9.2 billion, of which $6.8 came from Medicare (Medicare Payment Advisory Committee, 1998). The Balanced Budget Act of 1997 directed the Medical Payment Advisory Committee to study and make recommendations on federal policies supporting teaching hospitals and GME by August 1999. Part of the mandate includes evaluating federal policies regarding the methods for promoting the appropriate number, mix, and geographical distribution of physicians and other health professionals.

While there is an oversupply of physicians and nurses for personal health care, that is not the case in public health. Several studies have examined public health education and found significant shortages of professionals and academic faculty in a variety of public health fields (Harmon, 1996; Health Resources and Services Administration, 1992; O'Neil, 1993). The most substantial shortages were in epidemiology, biostatistics, environmental and occupational health, public health nutrition, public health nursing, and preventive medicine.

These and other concerns led the Assistant Secretary for Health in 1993 to commission an evaluation of PHS activities in training and education for public health (Harmon, 1996). The resulting report estimated that in fiscal year 1993, PHS spent $1.2 billion on training, of which $217 million (18 percent) went to training and education in public health, such as to schools of public health. The report found shortages in many fields and concluded that training and education in public health should become a top priority for PHS and that it should substantially redirect training support from biomedical research and curative specialty care to public health training and education. The report recommended expanding PHS trainee positions, especially in those fields reporting significant shortages. In response, DHHS released *The Public Health Workforce: An Agenda for the 21st Century* (1997c), which provided specific action items representing essential first steps in addressing the needs of the workforce for the new millennium. No action has been taken on the report at the time of this printing.

*In the future a logically integrated health information system will be needed – one in which information once collected can serve multiple purposes.*

### Information Systems

We believe that among the most important new developments for clinical medicine and public health will be the creation and expansion of public health information systems. A review by Friede, Blum, and McDonald (1995) and a National Library of Medicine bibliography

(1996) provide excellent background for public health informatics.

Newly emerging information systems cover an expanding variety of needs for the public health community. The extent to which population-based public health can achieve its mission depends on the effective collection, analysis, communication, and use among decision makers of this health-related information. Monitoring the health status of the community begins with data collection and analysis. The information produced must also be communicated and used if other essential public health services are to be accomplished.

Lasker, Humphreys, and Braithwaite (1995) have analyzed three components in this process – data collection and analysis, communication, and related decision making. Currently public health agencies rely on at least nine types of data to meet their needs. These include: (1) vital statistics; (2) periodic health surveys (e.g., NHANES, HIS); (3) disease and injury registries; (4) behavioral risk factor surveys; (5) disease and injury surveillance; (6) programmatic data systems (e.g., categorical disease control programs); (7) practitioner registries; (8) health care utilization data; and (9) health expenditure data. Consumer surveys are likely to be added to the list soon. Unfortunately the result is a fragmented collection of information, with episodic data collection, redundancy, and a lack of standardization. Essential data often are lacking at the local or state level.

In the future a *logically integrated* health information system will be needed – one in which information once collected can serve multiple purposes. Such a system is essential to hold both public health agencies and health plans accountable. As identified by the authors of this analysis, the elements of an integrated health information system are:

- a standardized, multipurpose nomenclature for all health concepts;

- uniform standards for electronic data transmissions;

- unique identifiers for all "units" of interest, including individuals, providers, worksites, restaurants, wells, etc.;

- strong privacy protection; and

- appropriate data sharing.

As they explain, the potential role of the National Information Infrastructure (NII) in creating an integrated health information system is an important one:

27

*The NII can also provide the necessary infrastructure to develop integrated databases, support analyses of the data, and make better use of data.... If all of the systems involved in the network collect data using a common vocabulary, aggregating data [that has been] collected for different purposes becomes practical and the burden of recording and resubmitting similar information to fulfill additional requirements is reduced.*

Such integrated health information systems will serve to record essential data, educate and empower different groups about public health problems, and link them together to take effective action. They will be increasingly important in measuring and assuring population health *and* the health of individuals. They also provide the means to assure accountability.

Communication of health information will involve not only face-to-face communication, but telephone, radio, television, video, e-mail or other means in order to inform, educate, and empower individuals and the community as a whole about public health problems, issues, and potential actions. Because the targets are quite diverse and people's needs and capacity to absorb information are also diverse, multiple strategies must be used. Too often public health practitioners overlook the mass media (radio, television) and rely too heavily on written materials (brochures) to get out their message.

As television can help public health practitioners educate the public, it can also help practitioners educate each other. For example, CDC has used distance learning – via the Public Health Training Network's satellite communication to multiple sites – to provide educational programs to more than 400,000 public health practitioners. North Carolina has used distance learning methods to reach public health practitioners in every local health department in the state. Another noteworthy effort is the Information Network for Public Health Officials (INPHO), an award-winning, 13-state, CDC-supported effort to connect public health to the Internet and provide on-line access to information and data.

*Performance monitoring is essential to assure stakeholder accountability in both health plans and public health agencies by identifying the range of stakeholders that can affect community health, monitoring the extent to which their actions contribute constructively to the health of the community, and fostering collaboration between public and private entities.*

Information is essential for the assessment, policy-making, and assurance functions of public health. Public health officials may need data from multiple providers to diagnose a disease outbreak. Clinical practitioners need efficient access to prevention and treatment guidelines and the ways that they can be applied to individual patients and to patient populations. Managed care plans and providers need data about the health status of their own populations, unmet needs, and organizational performance. Consumers depend on reliable information, currently distorted by heavy advertising and promotion of products by manufacturers (tobacco, fast foods). Health plan "report cards" are more often used for promotional purposes rather than to educate consumers and improve their choices. Consumers will increasingly be demanding reliable information on health plans, including information about consumer satisfaction. Information is also essential for policymakers at all levels of government, and in all branches of government.

The importance of population-based data for performance monitoring at the community level has been stressed in two recent IOM workshops on *Using Performance Monitoring to Improve Community Health* (1996b). Performance monitoring is essential to assure stakeholder accountability in both health plans and public health agencies by identifying the range of stakeholders that can affect community health, monitoring the extent to which their actions contribute constructively to the health of the community, and fostering collaboration between public and private entities.

In 1997, DHHS launched Healthfinder to serve as a gateway World Wide Web site (www.healthfinder.gov). Healthfinder is a point of entry to the broad range of consumer health information resources produced by the federal government and its many partners, and it will help consumers get information more quickly and easily. DHHS developed this site in collaboration with other federal agencies that have health communications responsibilities. To date, its use has exceeded expectations. More than 1.7 million visits were recorded in its first year of operation, and the second year's growth is reportedly keeping pace with the growing number of Internet users. While the site is experiencing success, in general health information on the Internet is not of consistently high quality and can unfortunately be misleading. As the information infrastructure is built throughout the United States, it is important to ensure that both medical care and public health requirements are addressed. Information technology offers an opportunity to link the health of populations and the medical treatment of individuals more closely, to the benefit of both.

# Working with Community to Advance Public Health

Within the community, there are many private and public organizations with a vested interest in protecting and improving the health of community members. By working together, these stakeholders can organize their roles and coordinate responsibilities in community health, as well as address matters of shared responsibility and individual accountability for specific actions. The IOM study, *Using Performance Monitoring to Improve Community Health* (1996b), found it essential for stakeholders to understand the Evans and Stoddart health field model (1994), which presents the dynamics of many determinants of health, ranging from health care to genetic endowment.

Once stakeholders can comprehend the multidimensional nature of the determinants, they can devise a plan for dealing with diversity in values and goals, establish successful working relationships, and strive toward community health improvement. In this section, we will provide several examples of community partnerships that seek to improve community health by focusing on the determinants of health: behavioral, environmental, genetics, and access to medical care. *Medicine and Public Health: The Power of Collaboration* (Lasker, 1997) describes more than 400 collaborative initiatives involving medicine and public health, and is an invaluable resource for those wishing to develop this type of collaboration.

CDC also developed the *Principles of Community Engagement* (U.S. Department of Health and Human Services, 1997b) to provide public health professionals and community leaders with a science base and practical guidelines for engaging the public in community decision making and action for health promotion, health protection, and disease prevention.

## Priority Areas for 2000

### Health Promotion
- Physical activity and fitness
- Nutrition
- Tobacco
- Alcohol and other drugs
- Family planning
- Mental health and mental disorders
- Violent and abusive behavior
- Educational and community-based programs

### Health protection
- Unintentional injuries
- Occupational safety and health
- Environmental health
- Food and drug safety
- Oral health

### Preventive services
- Maternal and infant health
- Heart disease and stroke
- Cancer
- Diabetes and chronic disabling conditions
- Human immunodeficiency virus infection
- Sexually transmitted diseases
- Clinical preventive services

### Surveillance and data systems

*Source:* McGinnis and Lee, 1995

Conclusions about successful initiatives put forth in the document include:

- Community engagement efforts should address multiple levels of the social environment, rather than only individual behaviors.

- Health behaviors are influenced by culture. To ensure that engagement efforts are culturally and linguistically appropriate, they must be developed from a knowledge of and respect for the targeted community's culture.

- People participate when they feel a sense of community, see their involvement and the issues as relevant and worth their time, and view the process and organizational climate of participation as open and supportive of their right to have a voice in the process.

• While it cannot be externally imposed on a community, a sense of empowerment – the ability to take action, influence, and make decisions on critical issues – is crucial to successful engagement efforts.

• Community mobilization and self-determination frequently need nurturing. Before individuals and organizations can gain control and influence and become players and partners in community health decision making and action, they may need additional knowledge, skills, and resources.

• Coalitions, when adequately supported, can be useful vehicles for mobilizing and using community assets for health decision making and action.

• Participation is influenced by whether community members believe that the benefits of participation outweigh the costs. Community leaders can use their understanding of perceived costs to develop appropriate incentives for participation.

The CDC also identified community-based public health services as one of three major components that are essential to U.S. health care reform. Along with community-based services, the general health of the public depends heavily on clinical preventive services and policies that promote healthy lifestyles and reduce hazardous risks. Although public health agencies are striving to improve quality of life for Americans, they also are struggling to maintain control over medical care expenditures. Prevention programming has the opportunity to play a key role in this process with the increasing demand for such programs that combine community-based services, clinical preventive services, and social policies.

*The CDC also identified community-based public health services as one of three major components that are essential to U.S. health care reform.*

The costs and benefits of prevention programs have been studied and results demonstrate that cost-effectiveness will ultimately be used to combine prevention activities with medical care reform (U.S. Department of Health and Human Services, 1994). Although community-based prevention is not typically recognized as the responsibility of private health care organizations, a recent trend among leading managed care organizations is to become involved in such prevention activities (Lasker, 1997). This support of community-based prevention by private health care will increase as long as managed care organizations continue to form partnerships with public health agencies (Gordon et al., 1996).

# Federal Partnerships with a Community Focus

In this section, some examples of community partnerships with federal agencies are highlighted.

## *Interagency Food Safety Initiative*

President Clinton announced a new initiative to improve the safety of the nation's food supply in January 1997. The goal of this initiative is to reduce, to the greatest extent possible, the incidence of foodborne illness. The announcement was based on a plan developed by DHHS, USDA, and the Environmental Protection Agency (EPA). Goals were outlined to work with consumers, producers, industry, states, universities, and the public to identify additional ways to reduce the incidence of foodborne illness and to ensure that the U.S. food supply is the safest in the world. Congress provided limited additional funding for this effort in the fiscal year 1998 budget.

Despite advances in knowledge, new challenges continue to threaten the nation's food safety programs. These include new pathogens, new food products that have unproven safety records, huge increases in imported foods, and increasing antimicrobial resistance among foodborne pathogens. Achieving a significant reduction in the incidence of foodborne illnesses requires the cooperative efforts of public health and regulatory agencies at the federal, state, tribal, and local levels, as well as for all other parties responsible for and concerned about food safety. Partnerships range from those between public agencies and industry, federal agencies and state, tribal or local agencies, and public agencies and academic institutions. These partnerships will enhance communication and should be invaluable in leveraging the resources needed. The cooperative action spurred by the President's directive provides a clear example of public health actions initiated at the federal level that will reach the community level.

## *Brownfields National Partnership*

Across America's urban landscape, many industrial and commercial facilities lie abandoned, idle, or underused because their development is complicated by real and perceived environmental contamination. These brownfields (in contrast to greenfields – pristine lands more often sought for business development) often lie near communities that include a large proportion of medically underserved and economically disadvantaged citizens.

Underdeveloped brownfields plague low-income, minority, or otherwise marginalized communities because they feed the cycle of urban decay, residential segregation, community disinvestment, and adverse land use. Over the past few years, public and private agencies have begun to ameliorate the health, social, and economic impact of brownfields. Environmental remediation training, public dialogues on brownfields' problems and opportunities, and model redevelopment projects have culminated in the Brownfields National Partnership Action Agenda.

The Brownfields Agenda embodies four basic principles: (1) protecting human health and the environment; (2) enhancing public participation in local decision making; (3) building safe and sustainable communities through public/private partnerships; and (4) recognizing that environmental protection can fuel economic redevelopment.

### Partnership for Prevention

Partnership for Prevention was created to supply private-sector leadership and educational resources to existing organizations for achieving national health objectives. To steadily improve the health of the nation, prevention must become an integral part of an improved Medicare program (McGinnis, 1997). Partnership for Prevention supports *Healthy People 2000* national objectives and improvement in Medicare's coverage of preventive services, many of which were added to the Medicare program by Congress in 1997. Partnership for Prevention proposes a comprehensive prevention program which includes not only effective clinical preventive services, but also public health activities, community-based preventive services, and prevention-oriented social and economic policies. The program also points out opportunities, as Medicare managed care grows, to efficiently develop preventive services and implement community-based approaches for prevention.

### Children's Environmental Health and Disease Prevention Research Centers

The CDC, EPA, and National Institute of Environmental Health Sciences (NIEHS) of NIH established the nation's first federal research centers dedicated to studying children's environmental health hazards. These centers are to conduct basic and applied research in combination

with community-based prevention efforts. Their aim is to better understand the causes of environmentally induced disease in children and eventually to decrease their prevalence.

In April 1997, a federal executive order (Protection of Children from Environmental Health Risks and Safety Risks) charged federal health agencies to consider special environmental risks to children in their activities. The agencies invited scientists from across the country to apply for grants to establish Centers of Excellence in Children's Environmental Health and Disease Prevention Research. Each application was designed around a central scientific theme, specifically examining the role of environmental agents in children's respiratory disease, childhood learning, and growth and development. In addition to basic biomedical research, proposals had to include a community-based intervention research component.

For this initiative parent agencies allocated $10.6 million to fund eight Centers. The first work of the Centers will address two of the most important areas of children's environmental health – the causes of asthma and the effects of pesticide exposure.

The long-range goal of this program is to promote translation of basic research findings into applied intervention and prevention methods, thereby enhancing awareness among children, their families, and health care practitioners regarding detection, treatment, and prevention of environmentally related diseases and health conditions.

## Accountability in Public Health

In their 1994 *Blueprint for a Healthy Community*, NACCHO and CDC proposed a system for creating and maintaining a healthy community, a system that safeguards the welfare of citizens. As a governmental entity on the local level, health departments assume the responsibility of assuring the public's health. Local health departments maintain and improve healthy communities by providing for ten essential elements that range from promoting healthy lifestyles to preventing and controlling epidemics (equivalent to the Ten Essential Services listed earlier). To successfully provide these ten elements, local health departments must receive adequate funding on all governmental levels, and develop staff capabilities in the areas of health assessment, policy development, administration, health promotion and protection, quality assurance, training and education, and community empowerment.

During the past decade there have been efforts at the federal and state levels to develop performance measures, including:

• Healthy People 2000

• Government Performance and Results Act (GPRA)

• Assessment Protocol for Excellence in Public Health (APEXPH)

• Performance Partnership Initiative, proposed by DHHS, 1994

The *Healthy People 2000* **program** has pioneered the use of performance measures. *Healthy People 2000* analysis tracks public health progress in the U.S. since 1990. In some areas great progress has been made. In other areas, the nation has been losing ground. And in still other cases, data is not available or performance measures have been too crude to determine whether or not progress toward objectives has been made. The next generation of projects is *Healthy People 2010*, a health promotion and disease prevention plan for the nation that will promote healthy people living in healthy communities. Scheduled for release in January 2000, it prescribes a national action agenda to increase years of life and quality of life, and to eliminate health disparities.

To prepare for *Healthy People 2000,* DHHS forged extensive working partnerships with other federal departments, states, communities, scientists, health professional organizations, industry, insurers, and the American people to identify and discuss key health issues. The goal of this extensive effort was to achieve consensus on targets and objectives, and to formulate a list of leading health indicators. *Healthy People 2010* includes more than 500 objectives that focus on risk and protective factors and preventive interventions for reducing premature deaths and reducing or eliminating diseases and disabilities. It covers the entire spectrum of determinants of health and measures of health status.

A short list of leading health indicators was also derived from the complete set of *Healthy People 2010* objectives and indicators, to sharpen the focus on actions that need to be taken to achieve progress. The leading health indicators focus on physical activity, excess weight or obesity, tobacco use, substance abuse, irresponsible sexual behavior, mental health, injury and violence, environmental quality, immunization, and access to quality health care. These ten areas are highly associated with diseases and other conditions that account for a large proportion of premature mortality in the nation.

**The Government Performance and Results Act (GPRA) of 1993** required all federal programs to have performance measures in place by fiscal year 1999. The Office of Management and Budget has coordinated this process and is requiring performance measures in a number of public health service programs submitted as part of the President's budget. Congress enacted GPRA because it wanted more objective means of determining what works and what doesn't.

**The Assessment Protocol for Excellence in Public Health (APEXPH) project** is funded through a cooperative agreement between NACCHO and CDC. APEXPH is a tool designed for local health officials to (1) assess the organization and management of the health department; (2) work with community members and organizations in assessing the health status of the community; and (3) establish their leadership roles in the community. Since the release of the APEXPH workbook in 1991 (National Association of County amd City Health Officials and the Centers for Disease Control and Prevention, 1994), many state and local health departments, community organizations, hospitals, and others have undertaken the assessment process. In a random survey of local health departments by CDC/NACCHO, nearly 80 percent of respondents knew of APEXPH, and of those, over 37 percent reported they had used or were currently using APEXPH kits to assess their organizational capacity. NACCHO is now field-testing a new electronic version of the APEXPH approach.

**The Performance Partnership Initiative**, begun in 1994, was an effort by PHS to develop a performance-based system of accountability. The goal was to create a partnership between the federal government, state and local governments, and the private sector to create a shared system of accountability to improve the health of the American people. The Performance Partnership grants shared a set of common elements:

• Flexibility for states to manage programs without detailed federal oversight of the process, but with agreed-on objectives and priorities among the partners.

• Performance measurement, using health outcomes as the meter by which success could be measured.

• Consolidation of multiple categorical programs to reduce the number of separate programs and create the potential for integrative funding.

Programs like these foster increased use of collaborative, multiagency or organizational initiatives that involve both public and private sectors (including public health and medicine) to address complex health problems that cut across traditional boundaries, e.g., HIV/AIDS, teenage pregnancy, family violence, and tobacco use by teenagers. In the past, federal agencies focused on making sure that federal moneys were used only for the specified activities or targeted populations as specified in legislation. The focus was on how the money was spent rather than on the results. The new system of accountability shifts the focus to improved health outcomes rather than expenditures.

In a 1997 report by DHHS, *Progress in Developing Performance Measures*, a number of barriers were identified. Within some agencies, a move toward devolution of federal government responsibilities to state, local, and tribal governments impeded rapid progress. For all of the agencies concerned directly with public health and health care, the absence of baseline data and a data infrastructure presented a serious problem.

The principal tool currently available for measuring the performance of managed care plans is the Health Plan Employer Data Information Set (HEDIS). From a public health perspective, the value of HEDIS is its value in measuring performance of health plans in achieving population health objectives (e.g., immunization for two-year-olds). While HEDIS is useful for capitated, population-based managed care plans, it is not particularly useful for the much more common type of managed care, namely discounted fee-for-service provided through preferred provider organizations (PPOs) or individual practice associations (IPAs).

Other problems with HEDIS measures from a public or community health perspective are the gaps noted among the indicators, as reviewed by the Center for the Advancement of Health and the Western Consortium for Public Health. Too little attention is given to the individual's functional status or health-related quality of life measures. In addition, the behavioral and psychosocial aspects of illness are not well addressed. Moreover, health promotion activities are focused on clinical preventive services and do not include broader measures of community-wide interventions (e.g., tobacco control).

## Future Trends in Public Health

Changes in the public health infrastructure have implications for community-based public health. As the federal government downsizes, public health functions will increasingly be transferred from the federal level to the state and local levels. Creativity and leadership will arise from within the communities for those responsibilities once delegated to the federal government. Accordingly, the government will become more of a partner in public health activities than the ultimate resource. In this capacity, more public health benefits can be leveraged from a constant or dwindling federal fund, and local citizen participation in building healthy communities has the potential to improve health outcomes even further.

## Acknowledgments

The authors gratefully acknowledge the assistance of Edward Baker and Michael Hatch, Centers for Disease Control and Prevention, and Erinn Noeth, Christina Coll, and Susan Bradford, Office of Disease Prevention and Health Promotion.

## References

American Cancer Society. Amicus Curiae Brief in Support of Petitioners, Supreme Court of the United States, no. 98-1152, 1999.

Annas GM. A national bill of patients' rights. *New England Journal of Medicine.* 1999; 338:675-699.

Baker EL, Melton RJ, Stange PV, Fields ML, Koplan JP, Guerra FA, Satcher D. Health reform and the health of the public. *Journal of the American Medical Association.* 1994; 272:1276-82.

Barry M, Centra L, Pratt T, Brown C, Giordano L. *Where Do the Dollars Go? Measuring Local Public Health Expenditures.* Published by the Public Health Foundation, National Association of County and City Health Officials, and National Association of Local Boards of Health; 1998.

Breslow L. The future of public health: prospects in the United States for the 1990s. *Annual Review of Public Health.* 1990; 11:1-28.

Brinkley A, Polsby NW, Sullivan KM. *New Federalist Papers: Essays in Defense of the Constitution.* New York: W.W. Norton & Co; 1997.

33

Brooks EF, DeFriese GH, Jain SC, Kavaler F, Miller CA. Local public health departments and their directors in North Carolina and the United States. *North Carolina.* 1976; 37:293-8.

Deaver GEA. An epidemiological model for health policy analysis. *Social Indicators Research.* 1976; 2:453-66.

Duffy J. *The Sanitarians: A History of Public Health.* Chicago, IL: University of Illinois Press; 1990.

Eilbert K, Barry M, Bialek R, Garufi M, Maiese D, Gebbie K, Fox C. Public health expenditures: Developing estimates for improved policy making. *Journal of Public Health Management and Practice.* 1997; 3(3):1-9.

Evans RG, Stoddart GL. Producing health, consuming health care. In RG Evans, ML Barer and TL Marmor (eds.) *Why Are Some People Healthy and Others Not? The Determinants of Health of Populations.* New York: Adeline De Gruyter; 1994.

Fee E. The origins and development of public health in the United States. In W Holland, R Detels, and G Knox (eds.) *Oxford Textbook of Public Health* (2nd ed.). Oxford/New York/Toronto: Oxford Medical Publications; 1991.

Fogel RW. Economic growth, population theory, and physiology: The bearing of long-term processes on the making of economic policy. *American Economic Review.* 1994; 84:369-95.

Friede A, Blum HL, McDonald M. Public health informatics: How information-age technology can strengthen public health. *Annual Review of Public Health.* 1995; 16:239-52.

Gordon RL, Baker EL, Roper WL, Omenn GS. Prevention and the reforming U.S. health care system: Changing roles and responsibilities for public health. *Annual Review of Public Health.* 1996; 17:489-509.

Harmon RG. Training and education for public health: The role of the U.S. Public Health Service. *American Journal of Preventive Medicine.* 1996; 12:151-5.

Health Resources and Services Administration. *Health Personnel in the United States—8th Report to Congress: 1991.* Washington, DC: U.S. Department of Health and Human Services; 1992.

Institute of Medicine. *The Future of Public Health.* Washington, DC: National Academy Press; 1988.

Institute of Medicine. *Improving Health in the Community: A Role for Performance Monitoring.* Washington, DC: National Academy Press; 1997.

Institute of Medicine. *Healthy Communities: New Partnerships for the Future of Public Health.* Washington, DC: National Academy Press; 1996a.

Institute of Medicine. *Using Performance Monitoring to Improve Community Health: Exploring the Issues.* Washington, DC: National Academy Press; 1996b.

Krieger N, Williams DR, Moss NE. Measuring social class in U.S. public health research: Concepts, methodologies, and guidelines. *Annual Review of Public Health.* 1997; 18:341-78.

Lasker RD. *Medicine and Public Health: The Power of Collaboration.* Committee on Medicine and Public Health. New York Academy of Medicine; 1997.

Lasker RD, Humphreys BL, and Braithwaite WR. *Making a Powerful Connection: The Health of the Public and the National Information Infrastructure.* Report of the U.S. Public Health Service, Public Health Data Policy Coordinating Committee; 1995.

Lee PR. Keynote Address. *Bulletin of the New York Academy of Medicine.* 1995; Suppl. 2, 72:552-69.

Lee PR, Benjamin AE, Weber MA. Policies and strategies for health in the United States. In R Detels, WW Holland, J McEwen, and GS Omenn (eds.) *Oxford Textbook of Public Health* (3rd ed.). New York: Oxford University Press; 1997.

Lee PR, Paxman DG. Reinventing public health. *Annual Review of Public Health.* 1997; 18:1-35.

Levit KR, Lazenby HC, Braden BR, Cowan CA, McDonnell PA, Sivarajan L, Stiller JM, Won DK, Donham CS, Long AM, Stewart MW. National health expenditures, 1996. *Health Care Financing Review.* 1997; 19:161-200.

Lipson D, Naierman N. Effects of health system change on safety-net providers. *Health Affairs.* 1996; 15:33-48.

34

McGinnis JM. Testimony before the U.S. Committee on Ways and Means, Subcommittee on Health. Washington, DC; March 13, 1997.

McGinnis JM, Foege WH. Actual causes of death in the United States. *Journal of the American Medical Association.* 1993; 270:2207-12.

McGinnis JM, Lee PR. Healthy People 2000 at mid-decade. *Journal of the American Medical Association.* 1995; 273(14):1123-29.

Medicare Payment Advisory Committee. *Report to the Congress: Medicare Payment Policy.* Volume I: Recommendations. Washington, DC; 1998.

National Association of County and City Health Officials and the Centers for Disease Control and Prevention. *Assessment Protocol for Excellence in Public Health.* Atlanta, GA; 1991.

National Association of County and City Health Officials and the Centers for Disease Control and Prevention. *Blueprint for a Healthy Community: A Guide for Local Health Departments.* Washington, DC; 1994.

National Library of Medicine. Public health informatics: January 1980 through December 1995. *Current Bibliographies in Medicine.* 1996.

O'Neil EH. *Health Professions Education for the Future: Schools in Service to the Nation.* San Francisco: Pew Health Professions Commission; 1993.

Rivo ML, Kindig DA. A report card on the physician workforce in the United States. *New England Journal of Medicine.* 1996; 334:892-6.

Rivo ML, Satcher DS. Improving access to health care through workforce reform. *Journal of the American Medical Association.* 1993; 270(9).

Rohrer JE, Dominguez D, Weaver M, Atchison CG, Merchant JA. Assessing public health performance in Iowa's counties. *Journal of Public Health Management and Practice.* 1997; 3:10-15.

Satcher D. Testimony before the Committee on Government Reform and Oversight, Subcommittee on Human Resources and Intergovernmental Relations, U.S. House of Representatives. Washington, DC; May 23, 1996.

Turnock BJ, Handler AS. From measuring to improving public health practice. *Annual Review of Public Health.* 1997; 18:261-82.

Turnock BJ, Handler A, Hall, Potsic S, Nalluri R, Vaughn EH. Capacity building influences on Illinois local health departments. *Journal of Public Health Management and Practice.* 1995; 1:50-8.

U.S. Department of Health and Human Services. *Surgeon General's Report on Promoting Health/Preventing Disease: Objectives for the Nation in the U.S. Public Health Service.* Washington, DC: Public Health Service; 1980a.

U.S. Department of Health and Human Services. *Ten Leading Causes of Death in the United States in 1977.* Atlanta, GA: Public Health Service, Centers for Disease Control and Prevention; 1980b.

U.S. Department of Health and Human Services. *Surgeon General's Report on Nutrition and Health.* Washington, DC: Public Health Service; 1988.

U.S. Department of Health and Human Services. *Healthy People 2000: National Health Promotion and Disease Prevention Objectives.* Washington, DC: Public Health Service; 1990.

U.S. Department of Health and Human Services. *Training and Education for Public Health: A Report to the Assistant Secretary for Health.* Washington, DC: U.S. Department of Health and Human Services; 1994.

U.S. Department of Health and Human Services. *For a Healthy Nation: Returns on Investment in Public Health.* Washington, DC: Public Health Service; 1995a.

U.S. Department of Health and Human Services. *1992-1993 National Profile of Local Health Departments.* Atlanta, GA: National Association of County and City Health Officials and Centers for Disease Control and Prevention; 1995b.

U.S. Department of Health and Human Services. *Surgeon General's Report on Physical Activity and Health.* Washington, DC: Public Health Service; 1996.

U.S. Department of Health and Human Services. *Progress in Developing Performance Measures.* Washington, DC; 1997a.

U.S. Department of Health and Human Services. *Principles of Community Engangement.* Atlanta, GA: Centers for Disease Control and Prevention; 1997b.

U.S. Department of Health and Human Services. *The Public Health Workforce: An Agenda for the 21st Century.* Washington, DC: Public Health Service; 1997c.

U.S. Department of Health and Human Services. *Surgeon General's Report on Health Promotion and Disease Prevention.* Washington, DC: Public Health Service; 1997d.

U.S. Department of Health and Human Services. Incidence of foodborne illnesses: Preliminary data from the Foodborne Disease Active Surveillance Network (FoodNet) – United States, 1998. *Morbidity and Mortality Weekly Report.* 1999; 48:189-94.

U.S. Department of Health and Human Services (DHHS/PATCH). *Planned Approach to Community Health: Guide for a Local Coordinator.* Atlanta, GA: Centers for Disease Control and Prevention. (Undated)

**Editors' Note:** *Quinton Baker outlines principles for engaging communities as informed, committed partners based on his experience with the Community-Based Public Health Initiative in North Carolina. Although the health challenges and opportunities he describes are specific to rural communities, similar examples could be provided from urban and suburban communities at a variety of socioeconomic levels. All communities have assets and issues. The secret to successful community-based partnerships is drawing upon the firsthand knowledge, energy, and interest of community members to identify and implement practical solutions within the community's unique cultural context.*

| Chapter IV | # Community-Based Public Health: The Community Perspective |
|---|---|

*Quinton E. Baker*

## Rural Poverty and Health

### Minnie Jane Faust

The winding dirt road lopes through tight mountains, rising past hog pens, cow pastures, goldenrod and honeysuckle, finally petering out at the home of Minnie Jane Faust. Slender as a paper clip, she is there shooing away wasps from her porch. The road delivers Chris Fuller, a community health worker who travels 400 to 500 miles a week trying to nudge poor rural families into health clinics. "Minnie Jane, it's been ten years since your last Pap smear," Fuller says. "You gotta go."

Minnie Jane's ponytail wiggles as she shyly shakes her head. "I don't go to no doctor," she says. "If I ever did have something bad, I wouldn't have no surgery anyway. I think once you know, and they start stuff, it makes it worse. If I don't know what's wrong with me, it won't hurt so bad."

### Chubs Moore

Chubs Moore grabs a piece of split wood and heads back inside his little house facing the dirt road at the edge of town. He and his neighbors on the road are conspicuously on the other side of the city limits sign. The 88-year-old Moore enters his kitchen, where two space heaters keep the room warm. He got so cold last night that he awoke at 3 a.m. and started a fire in the kitchen stove. He explains that he is afraid to run the space heaters at night because of the threat of fire. The Moores have lived in this house since 1945.

In the kitchen his wife Mattie, now 80 years old, speaks of the difficulties she and the other residents face in this mostly black, low-income neighborhood. "We tried for a long time to get water," says Mattie. "They built an apartment complex, and we got city water. Then they promised that we would get sewage service, but it never came. That was 10 or more years ago." She is no longer able to walk to the outhouse located in the backyard. She has to use a bedpan, which Chubs empties out back. He lifts a slab covering an abandoned well and dumps in the excrement. "I used to take it across the road and put it in the weeds," he says.

Just above Mattie's head the ceiling has a large hole. The ceiling tiles are warped. She explains that it rotted out, so they set buckets and pans to catch the water when it rains. Today, the ice on the roof is melting, creating a steady drip from the ceiling. Two years ago, an entire section of a wall crumbled from water damage and her son-in-law from Philadelphia fixed it by nailing some planks in. The floor has also sunk in where the wood underneath rotted.

### Vernell Jones

Vernell Jones has diabetes, or to use her word, "sugar." After many years of treatment she still doesn't understand the nature of her disease, its long-term implications, or how to control it. Having "sugar" is so common in the family and community that she thinks it's just another part of getting old. She has no earthly idea about those numbers the doctor's talking about. When she can get to the doctor, he tells her she's doing fine. Her sugar level is down a little. Three months ago it was 260; this time it's 230.

The doctor will check it again at her next visit in three months. She wonders if she'll make the next visit. Transportation to the doctor is often difficult, if not impossible. She has to get her daughter or son to stay home from work to drive her the forty miles to the clinic. Most times, she just doesn't go. It's hard to ask her children to lose a day's work just so she can get her sugar checked. They won't get paid for the day, and Lord knows they need the money.

### Faye Dean Lucas

North Carolina's Southern Orange County is dominated by Chapel Hill, the town nicknamed "the Southern Part of Heaven" with million-dollar homes and a world-class university. Chapel Hill produces high-powered medical specialists and sophisticated new biomedical interventions. According to *Money* magazine in 1994, this area was the "Best Place to Live in America." In Northern Orange County, less than 20 miles from Chapel Hill, Faye Dean Lucas loads the hatchback of her Chevette with empty plastic milk jugs. She drives to a gas station two miles away to fill the jugs with water. She uses the water to bathe, flush her toilet, and cook her family's food. Her mobile home has faucets in the kitchen and bathroom, but they're useless. The house has no water connection.

Her neighbor's septic tank constantly fails. Wastewater bubbles up in the vacant lot between their homes and flows down into Faye Dean's front yard, creating a smelly mess. It sits there for couple of days until the sun dries it up. She has a hard time keeping the children from playing in it.

## Medical Science and the Rural Dilemma

In these small houses where the Bible is always open and bean seeds dry in cloth bags, residents are at great risk for health problems. They make their own soap, kill rattlesnakes under the porch, pick off dog ticks every night, and share hand-me-down remedies for "what ails" them. Most will visit a doctor only if it's a dire emergency or if they are suffering from a lot of pain. Many share Minnie Jane Faust's reluctance to visit a doctor. "It just don't feel right going to the doctor," Faust says. "I just don't like the hassles they give you. Take this pill or that pill, but they never really tell you what's wrong. I'd have to be dying sick to go."

In many communities there is a pervasive strand of cultural fatalism; individuals don't see the need for medical checkups and services because "when your number's up, you're going." Or "it's God's will and there ain't nothing I can do about it but pray and trust the Lord." Many of these impoverished individuals are uninsured or underinsured. Those who do have insurance often lack the know-how necessary to use the health system properly.

Case files of health care workers and community organizers swirl with disturbing images: the eight-year-old boy who has dog food in his pockets because his family ran out of money; the little girl with pertussis who did not get the required immunizations; the low birthweight baby of a teenage mother who didn't survive; the uninsured mother who can't afford to have lumps removed from her breasts; and scores of men and women who die too soon from the end results of hypertension, diabetes, heart disease, stroke, and cancer.

Poverty and isolation are dominating issues, and they have rural people everywhere (including many low-paid health workers) wrestling with concerns much more basic than CAT scans, radial keratotomy, organ transplants, and medical reimbursements. If there's no food on the table, women can't really think about when their next Pap smear ought to be. Community health workers, like Chris Fuller, have no option but to help families with food, clothing, toothpaste, bathtubs, housing, and companionship if the ultimate aim is to urge them to take care of a long-standing ailment or schedule a medical checkup.

Despite the best efforts to achieve healthier families and communities, community health programs based primarily on a biomedical model fail to achieve their goal of improved health status in these neighborhoods. There is growing evidence that increases in the availability of medical professionals and services do not result in improved health status. Victor Fuchs has looked at this issue and concluded, "The greatest current potential for improving the health of the American people is to be found in what they [the people] do or don't do, to and for themselves" (1990, page 59).

*Despite the best efforts to achieve healthier families and communities, community health programs based primarily on a biomedical model fail to achieve their goal of improved health status in these neighborhoods.*

## Seeking Community Participation

Over the last decade, the concepts of empowerment, community empowerment, and community competence have captured the imagination of public health workers and community developers. In 1978 the World Health Organization (WHO) spelled out for the first time the importance of community participation in primary health care. More recent statements on health education directly link community participation to empowerment and such empowerment to healthier individuals and environments. Both medical and public health goals seem more possible when community people are empowered to participate actively in the health building process. Community *competence* (defined as a community's ability to collaborate effectively in identifying problems and finding solutions) has been associated with improved health outcomes. Both of these concepts seem to be health *enhancing.* The notion of involving the community is drawing attention as an important principle in addressing health problems, and word has begun to filter down to local levels through international and national health agencies and other groups.

Yet when it gets to the local level, the concept all too commonly is not well understood. Health professionals have had little, if any, experience with the process. A common scenario is this one: Because of governmental or other funding requirements, the community is requested to express its support and participation in interventions that health experts determine to be important and necessary. A few focus groups are set up and a town meeting of local residents is held at which the problem and its terrible outcomes are presented. This is followed by a glowing announcement of the intervention program that the department is establishing in the community to combat this terrible situation. The meeting concludes with a fervent request for residents to participate in the effort by joining the department to implement this "vital" new program that will benefit them and their community so much.

Such an approach is rarely successful, and it holds significant potential to further alienate the community it is intended to serve. Even the health professionals find the process frustrating. Not only do they fail to engage community groups in meaningful ways, they continue to assume that scientific progress in and of itself is sufficient reason for people to buy into the process. When rural residents don't participate in their well-intended programs, the professionals become dismayed.

From the resident's perspective it is all very clear: health professionals approach community people with issues and concerns that they have determined to be serious problems. These experts also delineate the best interventions for the problems. And over and over these interventions fail to alter significantly the health status of communities or residents. The explanation, of course, is that no matter how serious the problem is and the tragic outcomes might be, these issues simply are not viewed as priority concerns by the local residents. The basic necessities of life are much greater worries.

In addition to the attention factor, there are many cultural barriers that prevent people from addressing health problems. These include:

- Worry about loss of personal control during a period of treatment by doctors in hospital settings.

- Worry about imposing on children or others.

- Concern about loss of property or possessions while one is away from home.

- Inability to understand medical diagnoses and therapeutic instructions, which leads to embarrassment, anxiety, and avoidance of further contact with professionals.

- Pride that will not allow one to undergo therapy when there is no money to pay.

- Fear that a cancer diagnosis is a death sentence, since friends and relatives who have had the disease have died.

- Belief that illness is an indication of a morally and spiritually bankrupt life, and that God will heal illness when He is ready to do so.

- A perception that if one has a disease it is better not to know.

- A taboo against touching and examining the breasts or genitalia.

The real question is *whose* agenda is it, and *who* has decided that intervention is warranted or that a particular strategy is best for a given community or person?

## Authentic Community-Based Approaches

An alternate approach is certainly conceivable. If having outside "experts" intrude into unique neighborhoods is undesirable, particularly when they bring canned solu-

39

tions that are not locally understood or desired, what are the options? This book is about one such approach, as carried out in many different community settings. It is an approach that lets local residents work as *partners* with health and academic professionals to identify and address the issues that are important to their own community. The community-based public health approach shifts the mind-set away from providing community *services,* to building community understanding and capacity. Inherent in this shift is the move away from professional domination of health systems to a greater reliance on community engagement in problem solving and active collaboration.

The concept of community *capacity* asserts that local residents have sufficient resources in their lives "to cope with life's demands and not suffer ill-health effects" (Wallerstein, 1993). It is about groups of residents who decide that they have the power to determine what the problem is, and how it should be approached or solved. It is about demanding that they, the local residents, become key actors in implementing any solution. It is about assuming personal and collective responsibility, and a willingness to commit to personal and collective accountability. It is about applying the concepts of democracy to community action in the belief that sustainable solutions come from within, not from without.

Capacity building starts with determining what resources the community has. This involves counting the community *assets* rather than enumerating, one more time, the deficits. The concept teaches that inherent assets ought to be sharpened and focused to build and strengthen the community, thus to tackle the identified needs. It assumes that whatever the issue or concern turns out to be that is a priority for action, local residents, not outsiders, are the key to long-term solutions.

Identifying the assets that are present is not easy at the outset. Many of these are hidden in an inability to use language effectively, in anxieties and fears of inadequacy. Or they lie submerged under cultural stereotypes. Sometimes the perceived needs and problems of a community are so overwhelming that the possibility is never recognized that there are assets that can contribute to successful solutions. When this happens, residents must first gain some control in their own lives if they are to begin the process of partnering with others

to share assets that they have not yet recognized.

Focusing on the assets of communities, however, should not imply that there is no need for additional resources from the outside. Rather, it suggests that outside resources will be much more effectively used *if* the local community is fully mobilized and invested, and *when* the local community defines the issues and the agenda for which additional resources are needed.

Most communities need more resources, not more services. Resources differ from services in substantive ways. One difference is that communities can define how resources will be allocated, since utilization can be negotiated and molded to the expressed needs, issues, concerns, and assets of a given community. Services are harder for communities to regulate, since they often must be accepted or rejected as offered. Services tend to create dependency, whereas resources help people become more self-reliant. Because communities have very little say about the delivery of services, they often fail to utilize them even when they're needed.

*The community-based public health approach shifts the mind-set away from providing community services, to building community understanding and capacity.*

When professionals see themselves as bringing resources to a community, and are respectful of the assets and skills that community members bring, the community can and will make those resources more effective in achieving desired outcomes. By guiding the utilization of those resources to respond to the particular needs of their community, community members are able to guide health professionals in using their knowledge and skills to improve health and well-being.

Health is about community and our lives together in community. Communities quite commonly define health much more broadly than most health and medical professionals do. "Those conditions by which people can be healthy," the standard public health definition (Institute of Medicine, 1988), is a comfortable one for most community residents. Their focus is on those conditions and circumstances that cause poor health, not just the diseases or the poor outcomes alone. The health issues listed most often by community members are rarely the issues that are mentioned by the experts. More and more, however, through partnerships and collaborations, community people are helping health professionals understand their perspective on health, and the role that community members can and must play in creating health.

40

## Chatham County Partners Take Action to Improve Public Health

An example of the community capacity approach is the Chatham County Coalition of the North Carolina Community-Based Public Health (CBPH) Initiative. Coalition members include representatives of local community improvement and development associations, the county health department, the community action agency, the cooperative extension service, a local community college, and the School of Public Health at the University of North Carolina in Chapel Hill.

Coalition members come together as equal partners to discuss their issues, concerns, and problems, and the assets they bring to deal with those problems. Together they determine priorities and strategies that might be initiated to address them. It falls to community residents to take the lead in determining the issues and strategies to address community concerns. Coalition members bring personal and/or agency resources that can be negotiated and used to support those strategies. This negotiated use of resources might include leadership training and development activities, the training of community members to carry out specific functions that traditionally have been assigned to professionals, or the provision of necessary funds and personnel. Whatever the resource, the critical factor is that the community through its members and associations must be an active participant in determining the issue, the solution or intervention, and how professional resources will be used in collaboration with the community.

There are some things community residents can and should discuss outside the Coalition, just as the local health agency, the university, or other partners have unique challenges that do not affect the other partners. Like solid friendships, trust is an essential ingredient of healthy, effective coalitions. As trust builds, partners find increased pleasure in being together, working together. Over time things which initially seemed of little interest to one partner or another become more important as partners share issues that seem only to affect a given partner directly. Friendly banter, shared confidences, and a growing interest and pride in the progress and well-being of fellow participants makes partners and partnerships stronger.

*The most successful collaborative thus provides common ground for asset trading and sharing between the different partners.*

## Equality Among Partners

Bringing people together from different socioeconomic and educational backgrounds is not easy and cannot automatically generate successful outcomes. CBPH community coalitions brought together people from different racial and ethnic backgrounds, different faiths, different customs and values, and different experiences. We had vastly different perspectives of power and its uses. Our communication and social interactions were often tailored to our cultural and social backgrounds, and differed greatly in our ability to cross cultures. All who started on the journey had some level of trepidation about a social experiment of such far-reaching nature. What made it a success was our willingness to remain at the table together and learn from each other; to work through our fears and distrust by admitting that they were present and influenced the way we viewed each other and our motivation.

Together, we learned to recognize and accept that each partner brings to the process contributions that are very different, but of equal value for healing the community. What kept the process going was that a common problem ultimately was identified, and each group was dependent on the help of the others to solve that problem. It became a group with respect for each other and the contribution each makes – a derived interdependency, if you will.

This is a major paradigm shift. In this new scenario, residents are community members who are capable of determining priorities and solutions, as opposed to clients who need the professional interventions of others to solve their problems. They have the ability to join together with others to find solutions to the problems they determine to be important to their individual and collective lives. They negotiate for resources that might be available from other partners to assist them or strengthen their ability to change and improve their quality of life.

In this new approach, institutions, agencies, and professional caregivers must become more open, recognizing that communities have inherent capacity and bring unique assets. These assets can contribute to finding long-term solutions, not only for community problems, but for the institution's own set of problems. The most successful collaborative thus provides common ground for asset trading and sharing between the different partners.

# Jordan Grove's Diabetes Coalition

Some years ago, Jim Larson nursed his wife, bathed her sores, cooked her meals, and made sure that she did all that the doctor said to do before and after her dialysis. Jim's wife had diabetes and suffered from kidney failure as well as other complications of the disease. Jim knew that his wife had "sugar," and though he didn't really understand the problem he did recognize that his wife was very, very sick. He had learned that she was not supposed to eat foods containing refined sugar.

Jim Larson lives in Jordan Grove, one of the small rural CBPH communities. It is a close-knit neighborhood where most of the 156 residents are family members or close friends. Two years ago, concerned about the amount of illness in the area, the residents of Jordan Grove decided to do a community self-assessment. In collaboration with other members of the Chatham County Coalition, they developed a questionnaire to explore current health status and family health history. The community was surprised to learn that 46 percent of its residents have diabetes, but absolutely stunned to learn that 94.5 percent have relatives with the disease.

With this information, the residents decided to explore what might be done about the problem. Members of the Coalition and community members joined together to develop an eight-week training and information program. The community members who participated then developed their own group, the Diabetes Coalition, and now they work to help other community members understand what it means to have and manage the disease.

The Diabetes Coalition, in collaboration with the Chatham County Coalition, has established a diabetes self-monitoring center. The center offers residents with diabetes a place to monitor their glucose levels, on a daily basis if necessary, and an opportunity to gain the support of others in making necessary lifestyle changes. Community members staff the self-monitoring center under the guidance and support of the health department. In addition, the Diabetes Coalition sponsors potluck meals that feature foods prepared in a manner consistent with appropriate diabetic nutrition. Coalition members can invite family, friends, and others to share these meals.

The impact of this community-driven effort can be seen in Marlene, a woman in her late fifties who has lived with diabetes for more than 20 years. Recently, for the first time in memory, her blood glucose reached a normal level of 120. And Hazel, another lady in her mid-seventies and beginning to experience some of the long-term complications of diabetes, has said that she now understands the nature of the disease that has plagued her these many years.

These interventions were about a community discovering a health problem that was important for its residents and deciding to do something about that issue. The effectiveness of the approach reflected the ability of community residents to negotiate resources and partner with others who brought different resources to find a set of solutions that was right for this community. Most importantly, the community was able to own the problem from its own research and efforts. No one told the residents there was a major problem of diabetes; they discovered it through their own learning process. The community self-health assessment made joint and local ownership of the problem possible. Had the county, the state, or other outside professionals provided the same data, ownership would have been minimal. The community's capacity to carry out these activities and capitalize on new partnerships with academics and local health practitioners was thus a major determinant in allowing residents to assume responsibility for their own well-being.

Community capacity building is a slow and sometimes tedious process that requires much patience and commitment. Trust and listening are two essential and interrelated aspects. Trust comes with a willingness to listen, to set aside personal or institutional agendas to work on those issues and solutions that have been identified by the community. Listening means hearing those things that community members speak about with passion, both directly and indirectly.

In his book, *The Careless Society: Community and Its Counterfeits,* John McKnight reminds us: "Each of us has a map of the social world in our mind and the way we act, our plans and opinions are the result of that map. The people who make social policy also have social maps in their minds. They make plans and design programs based upon their maps" (1996, page 161).

Communities also have social maps. A fundamental question is whose map will be used to identify problems or goals, mobilize resources, and develop and implement strategies? Many professionals and institu-

*Community capacity building is a slow and sometimes tedious process that requires much patience and commitment. Trust and listening are two essential and interrelated aspects.*

42

tions tend to see vulnerable populations and communities as deficient, half-empty. As social and health policy mapmakers, do we build upon such a perception of emptiness? Do we create models based upon need? Or do we build assets and capacity, facilitating a process whereby communities use their voice to define their health concerns and solutions?

Community-based public health is a process through which communities in partnership with others identify common issues, problems, or goals. Then, they mobilize resources and develop and implement strategies for solving the problems to reach the goals that have been collectively established. The health professional's role is to help create the conditions in which communities, rather than outside experts, can determine and set the health agenda. Together they can begin to make a powerful impact on promoting health and transforming the lives of people in communities.

# References

Fuchs V. A tale of two states. In P Conrad and R Kern (eds.) *The Sociology of Health and Illness: Critical Perspectives.* New York: St. Martin's Press; 1990.

Institute of Medicine. *The Future of Public Health.* Washington, DC: National Academy Press; 1988.

McKnight J. *The Careless Society: Community and Its Counterfeits.* New York: Basic Books; 1996.

Wallerstein N. Empowerment and health: The theory and practice of community change. *Community Development Journal.* 1993; 28(3): 218-27.

World Health Organization. *Health for All: Declaration of Alma-Ata.* Report on the International Conference on Primary Health Care; 1978.

43

*Editors' Note: One major objective of the Community-Based Public Health (CBPH) Initiative was developing models to recast public health education, making it more practice- and community-oriented. As a result, some of the most remarkable changes that occurred through the initiative – those perhaps with the greatest potential for long-term impact – came about in schools of public health. In this chapter, one CBPH team reviews the differences between simply placing students into community settings for formal training and taking a systems approach to increasing the competency of graduates by promoting the principles and practice of community-based public health.*

# Chapter V | The Educational Perspective

*Lewis H. Margolis, Rachel Stevens, Barbara Laraia, Alice Ammerman, Chris Harlan, Jan Dodds, Eugenia Eng, and Margaret Pollard*

Recognizing the increasing complexity of the determinants of health and well-being for individuals and populations, many prominent groups have argued for changes in the nature of the teaching and research that constitute the educational experiences for students pursuing health and human service careers. The Pew Commission on Health Professions has urged health schools to focus on edu cation "that understands and serves a broader set of community needs" (O'Neil, 1993, p. 18). The Sun Valley Forum and the Association of Academic Medical Centers called for universities and health departments to "foster and participate in true collaborative partnerships and share responsibility in the development and implementation of a community-driven agenda to improve the health of the people and the health of communities" (Hogness, McLaughlin, and Osterweis, 1995, p. 169). In social services, the importance of collaboration and partnership has also stimulated interest in education on community building and practice (Morrison et al., 1997; Weil, 1996).

Reaching consensus, however, on the changes needed in education to bring communities to the center of the academic endeavor, whether in public health or other service professions, is fraught with difficulty. The purpose of this chapter is to describe the experience of the North Carolina Community-Based Public Health Initiative in addressing the issue of how to define and structure learning experiences – to enhance the competencies of students to practice public health in ways that foster collaborative partnerships with com-

munities. While many academic courses may expect or require a student experience "in the community," it is important to define what is meant by a community experience. The focus of this article is twofold. First, we define principles that underlie the term "community-based," in contrast to other types of community experiences. Second, we describe criteria to characterize courses and other learning experiences, in order to assess the extent to which they are community-based.

## Background on the North Carolina Community-Based Public Health Initiative

In 1992, the W.K. Kellogg Foundation launched the Community-Based Public Health (CBPH) Initiative and supported consortia in seven states to enhance the capacity of partnerships among community-based organizations, health agencies, and schools of public health to address public health issues (Parker et al., 1998; Margolis et al., 1996). The North Carolina initiative is built upon a set of principles to focus teaching, practice, and research in order to bring communities to the center of the public health endeavor. These principles emerged from an agreement among three community-based organizations, six health agencies, and two academic centers in North Carolina on conditions for joining a consortium to participate in this initiative. These conditions included, among others, the specification of particular community partners (instead of "community" as a setting), a commitment to community-identified issues and priority setting, and a

This article is to be published in an upcoming issue of the *Journal of Community Practice* under the title "Educating Students for Community-Based Partnerships."

focus on improvements in service systems rather than on addressing a categorical disease.

The first principle was that community-based public health enhances the capacity of communities to address issues of concern. Moving away from a service model that characterizes communities with needs and public health professionals as experts with the knowledge and expertise to address those needs, community-based public health strives to assure that community voices are, in the words of one community member, "at the table." More specifically, this principle meant that communities would become partners in the performance of the core functions of public health – assessment, policy development, and assurance (Institute of Medicine, 1988).

A second principle of community-based public health was that the consortium would broaden the participation of vulnerable communities. Whereas the first principle advocates a key role for communities in decision making, the second principle focuses on communities that are traditionally underrepresented in decision making and, therefore, often underserved. For example, in this initiative, the four community partners were predominantly African American, representing communities with income levels and other economic conditions that placed them at higher risk than neighboring communities for poor health.

A third principle involved the development of skills among community residents in mobilizing resources to address community priorities. An important aspect of this attribute is the recognition that community members have multiple personal skills (for example, leadership and organizational skills) and belong to numerous formal and informal associations, such as service clubs and churches, that can be nurtured and brought to bear on issues of concern. Further, while agency financial and programmatic resources are often essential to address public health concerns, the assets of community members may make the difference between the success and failure of an initiative in a community (Saleebey, 1997; Kretzmann and McKnight, 1993).

In order to advance these principles, the CBPH consortium fostered an approach to coalition building, consistent with community building in social work practice, for which the outcome of improved community capacity would be as important as improved health (Weil, 1996). This approach included strategies to enhance the capacities of community partners to (1) participate in and lead efforts to inform public health policy discussions and implementation; (2) redefine health agency relationships with the communities they

serve; and (3) develop greater community orientation in academic teaching and research (Parker et al., 1998).

These strategies were implemented in four counties, whereby local health agencies, community-based organizations, and the School of Public Health and Area Health Education Center of the University of North Carolina were represented on four distinct coalitions. Each coalition served as the organizing force behind community-driven projects to address public health issues that would contribute to the goals and objectives identified by communities. The community-based projects implemented by one or more of the four coalitions were: a neighborhood drug patrol (one coalition); recruitment and training of lay health advocates (three coalitions); youth health education and leadership training (three coalitions); a series of workshops or roundtables for minority business owners (one coalition); construction or renovation of community parks (three coalitions); and a chronic disease task force focusing on diabetes (one coalition). How the lessons learned from these projects were disseminated to students of public health is described in the next section.

## Implementing and Assessing Community-Based Education at the School of Public Health of the University of North Carolina

As articulated by the Institute of Medicine's *Future of Public Health* report (1988), the growing complexity of public health behooves educators to expand traditional, narrow, discipline-based competencies to include the "understanding of how a particular discipline relates to the whole of public health, and an appreciation of the relationship of public health to social endeavor as a whole" (p. 157). The Pew Health Professions Commission identified many competencies for health professionals for the year 2005 (O'Neil, 1993).

Although the focus of the Commission was on clinical services, several competencies are applicable to public health and/or population-based practice. For example, the ability to "understand the determinants of health and work with others in the community to integrate a range of activities that promote, protect, and improve the health of the community" is a competency that speaks to the practice of public health and implies a community-based dimension (p. 8). Understanding the need to emphasize "primary and secondary preventive strategies for all people and help individuals, families, and communities maintain and promote health behaviors," similarly suggests a community-based focus (p. 8).

Based on these competencies suggested by the Pew Commission and the lessons learned from the CBPH Initiative, we have worked with our community and agency partners to develop the following competencies for students to learn from courses that can be characterized as community-based:

## 1. The ability to enhance the capacity of community members to serve as partners in the performance of public health core functions.

This competency underscores the high value afforded to the concept of partnerships in community-based public health. While courses may teach students "about" communities, a community-based course would enable students and faculty to leave skills with community members. Planning a health promotion program, running a community meeting, or recruiting community members to join an activity exemplify skills that will enable community members to continue to have an impact on their communities, even after the student course or project has concluded.

## 2. The capacity to identify underrepresented or vulnerable populations and to enhance their participation in the public health endeavor.

This competency also builds upon the concept of partnership. Populations well-served by public and private agencies may be more accustomed to interacting with the university than are individuals from underserved communities. Encouraging community participation in assessments, program development, and evaluation by underserved populations will advance the abilities of students, faculty, and community members to act as partners.

## 3. Skills for mobilizing community resources to address community-defined priorities.

There are two principle components to mobilization – collaboration and identification of community assets. Community-based courses would help students develop strategies to bring varied interests together. Skills in promoting collaboration among groups of diverse backgrounds and building coalitions are fundamental to community-based public health. Another component would focus specifically on resources. The conventional view of program planning has been to identify "needs" or "deficits" in communities and then try to find the resources, usually financial, to fill those

needs (Saleebey, 1997; Kretzmann and McKnight, 1993). One of the important contributions of community-based public health has been to begin to integrate the concept of community assets and strengths into the practice of public health (Parks and Straker, 1996; Ammerman and Parks, 1998). Community-based teaching would develop an appreciation of the assets that communities themselves can bring to bear on issues.

After student competencies that reflect community-based principles were defined, the second step was to design learning activities that would appropriately and effectively develop the desired knowledge and skills. Historically, education for health and other service professionals has involved a range of activities from conventional didactic presentations, to structured and supervised clinical encounters, to placements in agencies that are responsible for assessing and assuring the health of populations. Field study, both in public agencies and in community settings, is a key component of many masters programs (Community-Campus Partnerships for Health, 1997; Council on Social Work Education, 1994; Center for Public Health Practice, 1993; Sorensen and Bialek, 1991). Similarly, many students are required to perform internships, which enable them to commit blocks of time to a particular setting outside of the school. Volunteerism represents yet another type of experiential education. Many students are drawn to public health, for example, because of the value they place on community approaches to public issues, so it is not uncommon for public health students to volunteer their time in formal organizations with longstanding agendas for social action or informal associations that come together to address short-term problems or concerns.

To assess which courses and learning experiences have the potential to develop the competencies needed for the community-based practice of public health, we have developed a matrix that consists of six domains: course goals, partner, exposure, product, classroom, and disciplines. These grew out of discussions among community partners and faculty participants about their shared and differing expectations for students who undertake community classes and projects. As a starting point for characterizing courses and other educational activities of the School of Public Health, we have applied a 6-point scale to each of these dimensions, ranging from 0 (no community content) to 5 (community-driven content). What follows is an elaboration of these domains as shown in Table 1.

47

## Table 1. A Continuum of "Community-Based" Learning Experiences

| | 1 | 2 | 3 | 4 | 5 |
|---|---|---|---|---|---|
| **Course Goals** | Community-based competencies are mentioned in course goals and objectives | Strategies to develop community-based competencies are described | Strategies to develop community-based competencies are strongly emphasized | The development of community-based competencies are a central component of the course | Primary goals of the course are to develop community-based competencies |
| **Partner** | Primary Care Treatment Facility, e.g., hospital | Primary Care Prevention Center, e.g., community health center | Agency working with community members | Community group in coordination with an institution | A grassroots group, serving vulnerable populations |
| **Exposure** | In the "community" one time observe | In the community partial time, e.g., a section of the class | Frequent visits to the community | On-going regularly scheduled visits to the community | In the community full time in order to enhance partnerships |
| **Product** | A single presentation to community members | A student initiated report to be used by a community organization or institution | A report, tool, or educational material to be used by the community, developed with some community input | A report, tool, or educational material developed with substantial community input | A community-initiated product with sustainable value, reflecting an understanding of local assets, created in partnership with students |
| **Classroom** | Focus of class is community-based issues and work, but no time spent with community members | Course occasionally brings people of the community into classroom to participate | Course regularly brings people of the community into classroom to participate | Faculty and community members together develop and plan a course that includes regular community participation | Faculty and community members in partnership to teach an interactive class, integrating students from several departments |
| **Disciplines** | One faculty teaching community issues from the perspective of a single discipline | One faculty member teaching a multidisciplinary approach focused on community-based health | Joint teaching by faculty from at least two disciplines | Faculty from different disciplines structure a course with content from different disciplines | Faculty from different disciplines structure a course that goes beyond the parallel use of different disciplines to engage in multidisciplinary inquiry |

## Course Goals

This domain assesses whether a given course explicitly addresses competencies necessary for community-based practice. Although skills such as data analysis, policy analysis, or environmental assessment may be important for addressing community issues and are crucial for a well-educated public health professional, community-based courses would articulate the principles outlined above.

## Partner

The partner reflects the responsible and participating group or agency outside of the University. An agency providing primary health care could be a community site for community-based teaching. Although primary care most narrowly refers to personal medical care that provides first contact with the health system, with comprehensiveness and coordination, more broadly it encompasses attentiveness to community-driven needs and desires. Therefore, a primary care treatment facility in a hospital would be community-based if it could demonstrate a role for community members in the setting of priorities. Slightly further along the continuum would be agencies for which the primary mission is to meet the primary and preventive needs of a community. Examples include local public health departments and community health centers. The next step on the continuum involves community agencies whose primary roles would be outside of health, but whose activities ordinarily involve a fair degree of partnership with community members. For example, course activity that works with Head Start or Housing Authority Residents' Councils would address the public health aspects of those programs. At the end of the partners continuum would be grassroots organizations. In the North Carolina CBPH Initiative, for example, the community partner in Wake County was Strengthening the Black Family, Inc. Formed in 1980 for the single purpose of sponsoring an annual conference on issues of concern to African American families, this organization, through its volunteer board and staff, now oversees a Teens Against AIDS program, a community computer access program, and the Southeast Raleigh Center for Community Health and Development, established to house CBPH Initiative activities.

Courses or field work that involved a primary care facility would received a score of 1 on partnership. Courses engaged with community-based organizations, such as Strengthening the Black Family, Inc.,

serving vulnerable and/or underrepresented communities, would receive a 5.

## Exposure

The exposure dimension refers to the amount of time spent in the community. At a minimum, a community-based (or more accurately at this end of the continuum, a community-focused) course would require a visit outside of the classroom. While classes may involve teaching and other forms of participation by community members in university classrooms, the community-based experience would encourage students to venture out from the University. Currently, it is possible for some public health students to complete their masters training without leaving the classroom. Students in five of the eight departments of the School of Public Health are expected to undertake an internship or practicum outside of the University, but these placements do not necessarily require time spent with a community.

Courses that involve a visit to a community site would receive a score of 1. Courses that encompass an ongoing placement at a community site with a community-based organization would receive a score of 5. The *ongoing* placement reflects the idea that the ability to develop and enhance partnerships is most likely to come from the commitment of substantial time.

## Product

The third dimension of this matrix is the expected product. The creation of a product that is of use to community members is an essential attribute of community-based teaching. At one end of the spectrum this would involve a single presentation to community representatives about the issue or question under study. At the other end of this spectrum would be a community-initiated product created in partnership with students. For example, recently a community-based organization raised the issue of school busing as a barrier to the receipt of school health services for children. Since magnet schools had been created in the neighborhood in order to attract a more diverse student population, most of the children in the community in question attended elementary schools in other parts of the county. A team of students enrolled in a program planning course applied these skills as they developed a framework for community members to use to begin to inform school health policy discussions.

Another student fulfilled an internship requirement by working with the four CBPH coalitions to plan and produce a video documentary of the project. In sum, a product that is motivated by community insights, utilizes community assets, and enhances the capacity of the community would contribute to the acquisition of community-based competencies.

## Classroom

The fifth dimension reflects the position that community-based teaching would be most effective when community members are coinstructors. A course receiving a score of 1 would be community-based solely because of its focus, but not include any classroom interaction with community members. The next level would occasionally involve community members as guest lecturers invited by the responsible faculty member. CBPH initiatives in Baltimore, Oakland, and North Carolina have developed this type of "community" faculty. At the other end of the continuum, faculty and community members, in partnership, would jointly plan and teach an interactive class, integrating students from several different departments and backgrounds. For example, we have developed a course titled "Community Voices," which brings together students from public health, medicine, nursing, pharmacy, dentistry, and social work; faculty from several disciplines; and community members to address ways to promote community-University collaboration and to develop listening skills, in particular, to facilitate work in the communities. While there has been some degree of joint planning with community members who regularly participate in the presentations, this course would be accorded a score of 4.

## Disciplines

In order to demonstrate the value placed on partnerships and the need for multiple perspectives to address public health issues, courses should expose students to more than a single discipline. Ideally, such a course would be team-taught by faculty members with different types of training and attended by students from multiple disciplines.

## Applying the Community-Based Matrix to Courses

For illustrative purposes we describe the application of this community-based matrix to two courses. The first example, "Rural Health and Community Action," ostensibly a course reflecting community-based principles and practices, received a score of 14 of 30 possible points. The "course goals" included the development of community-based competencies, but for the most part the course focused on rural health in contrast to the community action component so the score was 3. The course involved interaction with rural health agencies, but not community groups, so the "partner" score is 3. The class required no time spent outside of the School of Public Health in rural settings, so the "exposure" score was 0. Students produce papers reflecting a rural health issue, but since community members were not necessarily involved in the definition of the product, the "product" score was 3. Community members and rural professionals were invited into the class so the "classroom" score was 3. Finally, since the class is taught by a single professor, based on that individual's own training, the "discipline" score was 2.

The second example, "Public Health Program Planning and Evaluation," required students to work in groups of 2 to 4 in order to define a public health problem and develop a program plan to address it. For this illustration, one student project called upon students to develop community-based competencies, but not as the primary goal of the course. The score for the "coarse goals" would be 4. Since the students worked with agencies engaged with community members, the "partner" score was 3. Students spent part of their preparation in the community setting, so the "exposure" score was 2. The "product" score was 2 because the students defined the issue and produced a final report, without a required or expected community role. The "classroom" dimension received a score of 2 because community members were occasionally called upon to offer their expertise in the teaching of the course, in contrast to simply providing information about the issue in question. The "discipline" score was 5 because the course was team-taught by four faculty from at least three different disciplines, and involved students from as many as 8 departments. The total score was 18.

During the assessment process, it became apparent that more intensive analysis would be necessary to assign valid and reliable scores. For example, course descriptions, designed for informational and perhaps marketing purposes, did not always reflect the substance of courses at the level required for this analysis. Ongoing work will involve interviews and interaction with faculty members and students about the degree to which courses manifest these dimensions of "community-basedness."

## Discussion

As faculty in academic professional programs, we have come to recognize that community partnerships are fundamental to the practice of public health, social work, and other human services. As members of communities and lay organizations, we have heightened our expectations for academic professional training to transfer skills that enhance partnerships with communities. Through implementing our Community-Based Public Health Initiative, we have articulated three underlying principles of community-based work and defined three competencies that are important for students (as well as members of the service professions) to learn to develop partnerships. These competencies – understanding the importance of community capacity building, appreciating the role of participation by vulnerable populations, and developing skills for mobilizing community resources – give rise to more creative ways of thinking about curricula and criteria for accrediting professional degree programs.

To assess courses and other learning experiences guiding students in developing their capacities for community-based work, we have delineated six domains, each representing a continuum from minimal to maximal community-based focus. This tool may help to clarify for students, community preceptors, and faculty advisors what community-based academic training should accomplish. For example, learning contracts signed by three parties could define respective expectations, roles, products, and time commitments. Furthermore, such a tool can be used to compare and contrast service learning courses across academic units within a professional school and even across universities, given that the terms "community" and "community-based" have gained such currency. The application of this six-dimension matrix to self-identified "community" courses in our School of Public Health, for example, demonstrated lower than anticipated scores overall, thus highlighting the need for systematic curriculum planning and implementation that prospectively recognizes the multiple dimensions of community-based course offerings and field practica.

Faculty and community partners working with CBPH are continuing to refine these dimensions, as well as to assess curricula based on them. With the Durham-based Center for the Advancement of Community Based Public Health, established as a result of the CBPH Initiative, we are examining if and how the accreditation of other professional academic institutions includes community-based practice criteria. As the demands for the development of partnerships among academicians, agency professionals, and communities continue to grow, it is incumbent upon professional schools to exercise leadership in (1) defining and identifying the skills needed to educate graduates who are competent partners in communities, and (2) developing the methods required to enhance those skills.

## References

Ammerman A and Parks C. Preparing students for more effective community interventions: Assets assessment. *Journal of Family and Community Health*. 1998; 21:32-45.

Center for Public Health Practice. *Practica: A Guide to Field Placements of Students from Schools of Public Health to Public Health Agencies*. Chicago, IL: University of Illinois; 1993.

Community-Campus Partnerships for Health. *A Guide for Developing Community-Responsive Models in Health Professions Education*. San Francisco, CA: UCSF Center for the Health Professions; 1997.

Council on Social Work Education. Curriculum policy statement for master's degree program in social work education. http://www.cswe.org/mswcps.html; 1994.

Hogness JR, McLaughlin CJ, Osterweis M. *The University in the Urban Community: Responsibilities for Public Health*. Association of Academic Health Centers; 1995.

Institute of Medicine. *The Future of Public Health*. Washington, DC: National Academy of Sciences; 1988.

Kretzmann JP and McKnight JL. *Building Communities From the Inside Out*. Chicago, IL: ACTA Publications; 1993.

51

Margolis LH, Stevens R, Baker Q, Brewer L, Reimer D, Sherman W, Lowry P. *Disseminating Community-Based Public Health Throughout Local Health Departments.* Presented at the annual meeting of the American Public Health Association, New York, NY; 1996.

Morrison JD, Howard J, Johnson C, Navarro FJ, Plachetka B, Bell T. Strengthening neighborhoods by developing community networks. *Social Work.* 1997; 42:527-35.

National Policy Task Force. *Final Report of the National Policy Task Force of the Community-Based Public Health Initiative.* W.K. Kellogg Foundation, Battle Creek, MI:1996.

O'Neil EH. *Health Professions Education for the Future: Schools in Service to the Nation.* San Francisco: Pew Health Professions Commission; 1993.

Parker EA, Eng E, Laraia B, Ammerman A, Dodds J, Margolis LH, Cross A. Coalition building for prevention: Lessons learned from the North Carolina community-based public health initiative. *Journal of Public Health Management and Practice.* 1998; 4:25-36.

Parks CP and Straker HO. Community assets mapping: Community health assessment with a different twist. *Journal of Health Education.* 1996; 27:321-3.

Saleebey D. Community development, group empowerment, and individual resilience. In D Saleebey (ed.) *The Strengths Perspective in Social Work Practice.* New York: Longman, Inc., 1997; 199-216.

Sorenson AA and Bialek RG (eds.) *The Public Health Faculty/Agency Forum.* Gainesville: University of Florida Press; 1991.

Weil M. Community building: Building community practice. *Social Work.* 1996; 41:481-500.

*Editors' Note: Community-based research is a powerful tool for joining community, public health practitioners, and academic researchers in a common pursuit. As participants in this process, community is no longer the subject of study, but one of the architects — designing and implementing research that expands the knowledge base and supports community objectives. In this chapter, the authors describe the development, implementation, and dissemination of a set of community-based research principles, and detail the lessons and implications for academic, practice, and community participants in public health.*

|  | |
|---|---|
| **Chapter VI** | # The Research Perspective: Development and Implementation of Principles for Community-Based Research in Public Health |

*Amy J. Schulz, Barbara A. Israel, Suzanne M. Selig, Irene S. Bayer, and C.B. Griffin*

## Introduction

The intractability of many public health problems that are associated with economic, social, and political inequities has contributed to a growing interest in linking public health research institutions more closely with the communities experiencing and addressing those problems. This increasing interest in community-based public health research is grounded in the belief that partnerships between researchers and community members can contribute both to the development of new knowledge and to the ability of communities to address their local problems (Institute of Medicine, 1988; James, 1993; Hatch et al., 1993; Vega, 1992).

In this paper we examine historical, theoretical, and empirical foundations for the development of partnerships between community members and researchers, distinguishing among several models of community-based research. We describe the development of a set of principles intended to facilitate community-based public health research. Finally, we examine challenges, barriers, and lessons learned in the development and early implementation of these community-based public health research principles, and discuss implications for community research and practice.

## Background/Context

Some of the most persistent public health problems in the United States are associated with systematic inequalities in access to social, economic, and political resources. One approach to addressing these complex social and health problems involves community-based research and interventions that are context specific and that engage members of the community in the process of defining and addressing local health concerns.

There is a long and rich history within public health of working within community settings, and a corresponding interest in probing the sometimes unwieldy relationships among research and practice (Steuart, 1969; Steckler et al., 1993). For example, research designs that emphasize the generalizability of methods and indicators across sites have distinct limitations for community-based practice interventions that are heavily dependent on the context within which they occur (Israel et al., 1995; Mittelmark et al., 1993). In an editorial examining the tribulations of intervention trials, *American Journal of Public Health* editor Mervyn Susser (1995) noted:

*A gap exists between the constricted hypothesis of a tightly designed trial and the question at issue in the population at large. Thus trials may not provide the truest reflection of the questions researchers intend to pose and answer. Still faith in the randomized controlled trial is so firm among epidemiologists, clinical scientists, and journals — not excluding this one — that it may justly be described as a shibboleth, if not a religion. Science, like freedom, dies of dogma; subversion is its lifeblood. We need a more rounded and complex perspective* (p. 156).

Community interventions have often failed to diffuse new ideas, change behaviors, or achieve long-term acceptance because such projects did not obtain the participant's inside understanding of attitudes, needs, and the environment (Elden, 1983, 1986; Paul, 1995; Steuart, 1975; Rogers and Shoemaker, 1971). In addition to being ineffective, community practice efforts that fail to engage participants in the design, management, and control of the research and intervention process may limit the extent to which communities develop the capacity to address local health concerns themselves (Elden, 1983; Israel, Schurman, and House, 1989; Fisher, 1995; Hatch et al., 1993). Recognition of these limitations has contributed to the development of research approaches that involve stronger relationships among community members, members of the public health practice community, and public health researchers, in order to facilitate exchange and collaboration (Steuart and Kark, 1993; Steckler et al., 1995; Marin et al., 1995; Clark and McLeroy, 1995).

The community-based research principles discussed in this paper were developed within the context of the Detroit-Genesee County Community Based Public Health Consortium (hereafter, the CBPH project), made up of representatives from community-based organizations, local health departments, and educational institutions.[1] The CBPH project was one of seven consortia nationwide funded by the W.K. Kellogg Foundation's CBPH Initiative. The intent of this effort was to bring together academic researchers, practitioners, and community-based organizations; to increase these groups' understanding of the connections among health status and social, economic, and cultural conditions; to better understand the relationship of community decision-making processes to health status; and to increase the responsiveness of health professionals, political and human service organizations, and community leaders to the health concerns of marginalized communities (W.K. Kellogg Foundation, 1992).

The community-based public health principles grew out of the efforts of the CBPH project to facilitate research processes that were responsive to, and driven by, concerns identified by local communities. They were guided by key elements of community-based approaches to public health research and education, defined by project members. These included:

• An emphasis on the local relevance and changing nature of public health problems which are shaped by the combined influence of the social and physical environment and cultural and psychological factors that influence health status and health-related behaviors;

• A commitment to enhance knowledge and promote change in ways that benefit the involved communities, student learning, and the field of public health;

• Building on, and strengthening, existing capacities within communities; and

• Developing multiple partnerships among the University of Michigan School of Public Health, local health agencies, health care providers, and community-based organizations in order to effectively study and address public health needs of the community, and enhance the relevance of the curriculum to local concerns.

These key characteristics of a community-based approach to public health reflect an overall orientation within the CBPH Initiative that encourages the integration of knowledge and action. The community-based research principles are consistent with, and seek to promote, this philosophy by increasing the participation and influence of community members in the process of generating knowledge about local health concerns, and linking the development of knowledge or theory with action to address those concerns.

## Theoretical/Conceptual Basis

Participatory forms of research have their foundation in theoretical frameworks that recognize that knowledge is socially constructed and a form of power, and that knowledge connected to lived experience trans-

[1] Partners involved with the Detroit-Genesee County CBPH project included: Barton McFarlane Neighborhood Association; Chi Eta Phi Sorority; Coalition for Positive Youth Development; Community Police Relations Committee, Precincts 2 and 12; Detroit Health Department; Flint and Vicinity Coalition for Economic Development; Flint Neighborhood Coalition; Flint Odyssey House; Genesee Area Skills Center; Genesee County Community Action Agency; Grace Hospital; Hartford Agape House; Hartwell and Neighbors; Monier Elementary School; National Center for the Advancement of Blacks in the Health Professions; Neighborhood Service Organization; Pierson Elementary School; Sinai Hospital; The Special Institute; University of Detroit/Mercy; University of Michigan-Flint; University of Michigan School of Public Health; Wayne State University.

lates into action more readily than knowledge that is disconnected from practice. This perspective emphasizes the ways that knowledge – including scientific knowledge – is shaped by social and historical processes, the location of social groups in relation to each other, and the meanings and interpretations ascribed to events and experiences (Jaggar, 1988; Collins, 1990; Harding, 1991; Smith, 1987; Jaggar and Bordo, 1989; Fay, 1987; Henderson, 1994). This literature challenges the assumptions of Cartesian philosophies of knowledge, arguing that knowledge is not objective nor static, but always partial, value based, and continually evolving (Hall, 1975).

Some of these critical theorists have proposed that a more complete knowledge might be developed through dialogue among those who occupy different social positions, and who bring different perspectives and understandings. However, this knowledge will be shaped or distorted by social asymmetries such as those structured around race/ethnicity, class, gender, and sexual orientation in the contemporary United States unless they are recognized and explicit efforts are made to address them by, for example, creating processes which ensure the participation and influence of those who traditionally have less influence (Habermas, 1975; Harmon and Mayer, 1986; Collins, 1990).

Social, political, and economic inequalities can be reinforced or challenged through the representation of social groups in the knowledge-production process (Mulling, 1992; Feagin and Feagin, 1994; Collins, 1990). Budd Hall (1975), in an early critique, noted that the failure to include community members in the process of developing knowledge about their lives and the concerns they face both reflects and reinforces "the illusion that community members are unable to gather and analyze data themselves" and to act upon their interpretations of that information (p. 25-27).

In addition, research processes that do not involve community members may fail to learn from the lived experience of community members and their interpretations of those experiences, and may fall short in efforts to change power relationships that marginalize some communities (Hooks, 1984; Yeich and Levine, 1992). In contrast, frameworks that integrate theory and practice, that are connected with lived experience and linked with social change efforts, can contribute to the ability of disenfranchised groups to name their experience and act to create change (Hooks, 1984, 1989; Lewis and Ford, 1990; Gutierrez, 1990).

# Developing Alternative Frameworks

**Participatory forms of research.** There is a long and rich history of research in the social sciences that integrates the development of new knowledge with action (Bailey, 1992; Stoeker and Bonacich, 1992). As early as the 1940s, Kurt Lewin coined the term "action research" to describe the use of the social sciences to inform social and organizational decisions and actions (Lewin, 1946). Reviews of participatory and action research examine their use in the arenas of community organizing (Alinsky, 1971), agricultural extension education (Austin and Betten, 1990), community development (Stoeker and Beckwith, 1992; Fals-Borda, 1988; Frideres, 1992), and others (Stoeker and Bonacich, 1992). Within this long and diverse history, different forms of participatory research have developed, and some authors distinguish among "action research," "participatory research," and "participatory action research." In brief, participatory action research is often used to describe research that emphasizes both action and the participation of traditionally disenfranchised groups in the research process, and that includes an explicit analysis of power differentials and the need for structural change to address social inequalities.[2]

Participatory forms of research challenge the development of knowledge that is disconnected from people's lived experience, producing "collective, locally controlled knowledge which leads to action on problems directly and immediately affecting the participants … " (International Council for Adult Education, 1980). Research that involves those affected by the issue as active participants (not as objects to be studied) facilitates the creation of knowledge that is relevant to the questions asked by those who experience the problem and offers them opportunities to define potential solutions or actions. The involvement of community members recognizes the validity of active engagement, and affirms the capacity of community members to address their concerns. It can result in the development of new knowledge that is directly linked with action and social change.

Max Elden describes four critical decisions made in any research project: defining the research problem; developing the study design; analyzing and interpreting the data; and putting the findings to use (Elden, 1987). Participatory action research creates opportunities for those affected by the research topic to participate and to have influence in those decision processes. It does not prescribe a particular research design or type of

55

data (e.g., quantitative or qualitative), but rather suggests that decisions made about research questions and the methods used to gather information be determined in collaboration with members of the community affected by the research.

Participatory action research is not appropriate for every issue, but may be an effective approach when the research is concerned with developing knowledge that is informed by multiple perspectives, including the experience of those who are most affected by the issue, and when knowledge is explicitly linked to efforts to change social conditions that affect, for example, health status.

**Community-Based Research.** Research that is based or conducted in community settings may or may not use a participatory action research approach. In a recent article, Hatch et al. (1993) describe four models of community-based research. The first involves consultation by the researchers with human resource providers or other professionals who work in the community but who are "at the periphery of community cultural systems" (p. 28). The second model involves identifying key members of the community, explaining the research project to them, and requesting their endorsement of the project. In both of these models, the research is conducted in a community setting, but the role of the community in setting the research agenda is essentially passive. The principles and underlying assumptions of a participatory action approach to research are not utilized.

In the third model, the researchers contact key community members, explain the research to them, and "ask for support, guidance, and advice in hiring community people as interviewers, outreach workers, and screeners" (p. 28). The authors suggest that this model achieves greater community involvement, but notes the absence of structured opportunities for community members to influence the research questions, design, methods, or the interpretation of the research results.

The fourth model of community-based research, which the authors term "community/researcher partnerships," involves active community participation. The researcher seeks community assistance in setting the direction and focus of the research, defining the study problem, and constructing the research design: community members are collaborative partners in the research process. The assumptions that knowledge is socially constructed and that knowledge is a form of power are reflected in the development of participant/researcher partnerships, intended to both address inequities in more traditional research designs and to

create knowledge that incorporates multiple standpoints and interpretive frameworks.

Furthermore, such partnerships reflect the assumption that knowledge directly linked with the experience of community members is more readily acted upon by those who "have the right to be actively involved in the management of their destinies, and consequently to avoid becoming the victims of others' good (or bad) intentions" (Singer, 1993, p. 17 quoting Chamber, E., 1985). In addition to providing community members with shared ownership of the research process, community/research partnerships enhance the ability of community members to create change within their communities by bringing together their local knowledge with the new knowledge produced through the research process.

It is the fourth model of community/research partnerships that underlies the development of the community-based public health research principles by the Detroit-Genesee County Community-Based Public Health Consortium. This model of research is consistent with the key elements presented earlier of community-based approaches to public health research and education, as these were defined by the consortium.

# Development of the CBPH Research Principles

**Context within which the principles were developed.** The Detroit-Genesee County Community-Based Public Health Consortium was comprised of three teams: the Detroit team, the Genesee County team (also known as the Broome team), and the University of Michigan School of Public Health team. The Detroit and Genesee County teams were each comprised of representatives from community-based organizations, the local health department, and educational institutions, including the University of Michigan School of Public Health. The School of Public Health team was comprised of faculty representatives from each of the departments at the School, representatives from each of three schoolwide student organizations at the School, and representatives from the Detroit and Genesee County teams. Each team met regularly to discuss, plan, and make decisions regarding team- and consortium-related matters. In addition, representatives from each of the three teams met every other month as part of the Collaborating Group, the communication and decision-making body for the consortium as a whole. Finally, cross-cutting groups with representatives from each of the three teams were formed to address particular issues within the consortium (e.g., communications and linkages; evaluation; policy; and research).

During the first year of the CBPH project, members of the collaborating group were asked, in in-depth interviews, to discuss their vision for the consortium as a whole. Analysis of these interviews indicated that five broad goals were shared across the three teams and across the three types of organizations comprising each team (health department, community-based organization, and academic). The goals identified were:

Improve community health;

Develop collaborative relationships among the involved groups;

Promote change within and between the organizations involved with the CBPH project;

Increase the participation and influence of community members in addressing community health concerns; and

Inform local, state, and federal policy discussions related to community health.

The community-based research principles were viewed as a guide for the development of community/research partnerships that would, in turn, facilitate progress toward the following goals:

Foster the development of collaborative relationships among researchers and community members that would promote change within and between the organizations involved with the CBPH project;

Increase the participation and influence of community members in the process of developing knowledge about community health concerns; and

Provide information to inform local, state, and federal policy discussions related to community health.

**Process of development.** The Detroit-Genesee County CBPH project began in January of 1993 and by that spring, the collaborating group had received several inquiries from researchers who were interested in the organizations involved with the consortium as sites for research projects. A cross-cutting group on community-based research (hereafter referred to as the

CCG), with representatives from the Genesee County, Detroit, and School of Public Health teams, was created to develop a philosophy statement and set of principles and procedures that would be followed in conducting community-based research that was consistent with the overall philosophy and goals of the consortium.[3] Efforts were made to create a cross-cutting group that reflected the composition of the larger consortium, with representation across communities and across the three types of organizations involved with the consortium; however, there was overrepresentation from academic partners.[4]

In the spring of 1993, the CCG began a series of discussions about the potential for research within the consortium and ways to facilitate research that would address community concerns. The group developed a general philosophy statement that outlined the intention of the consortium to encourage research partnerships that would contribute to the ability of communities to address their health needs and develop new knowledge about the identification and resolution of public health problems. The statement was presented at a July 1993 meeting of the collaborating group. It was discussed and approved, and the CCG was asked to develop more specific objectives and principles.

Two months later, the CCG distributed an initial draft of the community-based research principles and procedures for implementing them to members of the collaborating group for review and comment. The principles focused on creating partnerships between researchers and those who were affected by the issue of concern, who would work together to define research questions and methods, interpret the results, and determine the mutual benefits of the research process. The CCG also developed a flow chart and procedures statement to provide a guide through the process, indicating whom to contact, and key questions to be negotiated in developing a research plan.

**Process of adoption.** At the recommendation of the collaborating group, each of the three teams reviewed and discussed this initial draft of the community-based research principles. The principles generated perhaps the most discussion at the School of Public Health's CBPH committee meetings, where they were on the agenda in both October and November, 1993. There

57

[3] Several of the authors of this paper were members of the cross-cutting group on community-based research.

[4] The cross-cutting group on community-based research was made up of three faculty members, representing the School of Public Health, the Detroit, and the Genesee County teams; one graduate student who was employed with the CBPH project, one of the two evaluators for the CBPH project, the project director from the Detroit team (employed by a community-based organization) and the project coordinator from the Genesee County team (employed by the local health department).

was relatively little discussion of the principles at the Genesee County team meetings during the two sessions in which they were on the agenda, and there was considerable discussion about several aspects of the principles over two Detroit team meetings.

Several issues were raised for discussion as team members sought to reach consensus on the community-based research principles that they would adopt. These included: (1) clarifying the definition of community-based research; (2) communicating the value of community-based research; (3) gatekeeping versus facilitating roles in creating community/research partnerships; (4) defining "ownership" of the research; (5) expediting the process of building community/research partnerships; and (6) distributing the principles. As described below, some of these issues were of greater concern to researchers than to community members (e.g., concerns about gatekeeping and access to community groups for research purposes) while others were of concern to both researchers and community members (e.g., "ownership" of the data).

**Clarifying the Definition of Community-Based Research.** Much of the discussion in the School of Public Health Team focused on clarifying definitions of community-based research. The phrase "community-based research" meant different things to different team members, from research conducted in community settings but without involving community members in the research process to models in which community members were explicitly involved in the research design and implementation. One team member, seeking to distinguish between these models and to emphasize that the principles promoted community partnerships and not research simply carried out in community settings, noted:

> There is a distinction here between doing research in the community and doing research that is community-based research. These principles help define *community-based* research.

Some faculty were concerned that the principles would invalidate research that was not conducted in partnership with community members, recognizing that such research might be equally or more appropriate for some types of problems or questions. In response, team members worked to define the parameters of the community-based research principles – to whom they would apply and when – as in the following excerpt:

> *These principles were created by members of the team from Detroit and Flint communities and the School, and apply to anyone wanting to do community-based research*

*(with the CBPH project). This is a different set of principles than traditional research in the community. With these, the community would decide what their role is in conjunction with the researcher.*

This process of dialogue and clarification both led to modification and clarification of the principles, and provided an opportunity for team members to grapple with real concerns that would arise as they sought to describe the principles to others.

**Communicating the Value of the Community-Based Research Principles.** A second issue discussed in these School of Public Health team meetings was that of why, and when, researchers or community members would wish to work through the process outlined in the community-based research principles. Several members of the team noted that following the principles would add steps to the development of research proposals and might slow down already short timelines. Furthermore, some faculty members were concerned that community groups might make requests that would interfere with the conduct of research, as in the following excerpt from the field notes:

> *What if a researcher goes into the field with some scales that have been validated elsewhere, that have validity that is proven – you don't want to have someone go through your scales and say "we don't want you to use this item or this item." Some things are nonnegotiable.*

Discussion about this concern focused on the importance of developing partnerships that allow for communication about issues of research reliability and validity; recognition of the real concerns that members of communities may have regarding research instruments; and the potential value of allowing research questions and designs to be shaped by those who are knowledgeable about the community. Furthermore, team members identified a number of benefits to researchers who elected to work with the CBPH project on community/research partnerships. These included: the assistance of CBPH project participants in identifying and facilitating linkages with members of the community of interest; increased community support for and participation in the project associated with improved quality and quantity of responses; improved effectiveness of intervention research; and potential benefits of basic research for the community.

While members of one of the community teams voiced few concerns about the principles or communicating them to others, members of the other team raised many questions about whether they or other members of their communities would benefit from participating in such a process. Some of these concerns are discussed in the section titled Defining Ownership, and highlight some of the questions of those who are not researchers about the value of participating in community/researcher partnerships.

**Gatekeeping vs. Facilitating Community/ Research Partnerships.** Some faculty were concerned that the principles, and as a result the CBPH project, might be perceived as screening or limiting the access of researchers to community groups with whom they might want to work, and limiting the types of research conducted. First, the CCG clarified that the principles were intended only to guide research that was conducted through the CBPH project, not all research conducted by researchers at the School of Public Health. Second, the CCG emphasized that the community members, not the School of Public Health's team, would be the researchers' point of contact for developing research projects consistent with the principles. Third, several members of the various teams clarified the role of the project coordinators in each community to facilitate research by helping to create linkages between researchers and community groups or organizations with a potential interest in the research topic. For example:

> The organizations involved in this project made a commitment to work in this way. It's not intended to be a gatekeeper in any sense of the term. The communities' commitment is to be involved in research as well as in other facets of the project, and we've negotiated a process of how this will be.

Finally, CCG members noted that the community-based research principles were simply principles, not directives or rules, and that they were intended to facilitate the development of community/research partnerships, not to eliminate other types of research.

**Defining Ownership.** One of the most contentious issues within the negotiation process was that of "ownership" of the research. Through the process of discussing the principles over a period of several months, one difficulty arose from differing meanings associated with the word "ownership." For many whose primary work was not research, ownership meant being able to participate and have influence in the process of defining research questions, and to have access to the research results to inform their work within the community. Many researchers were concerned about the physical

location of the data (where it would be housed) and control over access to it, the ability to ensure confidentiality to participants in the research process, and the ability to publish based on the research. Once these different meanings of ownership were clarified, language was developed in the principles that distinguished among them. Thus, the committee defined joint ownership more specifically as: working together to define research questions and methods; create opportunities for dialogue and reflection on the research results; provide community access to research findings; and involve community members in jointly authored publications.

**Expediting the Process.** Once again, this was primarily a concern of researchers, who pointed out that they often have a relatively short time period within which to write a proposal in order to meet set deadlines. There was concern that additional requirements, such as working through the procedures that accompanied the community-based research principles, might slow down the proposal writing process and result in some missed opportunities for funding. The benefits to the research of developing long-term relationships with community members founded on mutual trust and shared goals were discussed. Some School of Public Health team members noted that proposals developed on short timelines might not have the necessary stability of relationships that take time to develop. Given that many funding opportunities have recurring deadlines, members suggested that a researcher who noted a proposal of interest might initiate contact with community groups in order to establish a working relationship, with the intention of submitting a collaborative proposal at a later date.

Other faculty members of the School of Public Health team also pointed out that the Detroit-Genesee County CBPH project itself provided a solid foundation that might expedite the process of developing research partnerships. Relationships had been established among the community-based organizations involved with the project, the local health departments, and those faculty involved with the CBPH project which could develop into research partnerships. Finally, the project coordinators from the two community teams noted that they were interested in facilitating community/research partnerships, not in erecting unnecessary roadblocks. If they considered that the proposed research would benefit the community, and had the potential to develop into a strong research partnership, they were willing to consider an expedited process on a case-by-case basis.

**Distributing the Principles.** The community teams discussed dissemination of the principles among participating organizations and processes for communicating their purpose. Within the School of Public Health team, once again issues of for whom the principles were intended, and how they would be distributed, came to the fore. The team agreed that while the principles were to be made available throughout the school, they were clearly not relevant for all faculty nor all types of research:

> We're not trying to get the whole school to adopt these. We want to share them with faculty and generate interest in doing community-based research. There is not an expectation that all faculty will change the way they do research, but help facilitate it among those who might be interested.

Thus, dissemination to other faculty was designed to inform a broad range of faculty, recognizing the many valid forms of research that may not be compatible with these principles (e.g., laboratory research), and to encourage those with an interest to consider developing research partnerships with the organizations affiliated with the Community-Based Public Health project. A cover sheet describing the goals and objectives of the Community-Based Public Health project, the rationale behind the principles, and the philosophy of community-based research held by the CBPH project was to be attached to the community-based research principles before they were distributed.

After several rounds of revisions to address the above concerns, the final version of the principles was agreed upon by each of the three teams and formally adopted by the collaborating group in January 1994. A copy of the principles as they were adopted is shown in Figure 1.

**Dissemination of the Principles.** Following adoption of the community-based research principles, the next step was distribution within the CBPH project and beyond. Theories about the diffusion of innovations suggest that they are more likely to be accepted if they are presented by a credible member of one's own group (Rogers and Shoemaker, 1971), and the principles were disseminated in a manner consistent with this perspective.

First, each member of the consortium received a copy of the principles with a cover memo describing their purpose. In the Detroit and Genesee County teams, the project coordinators and members of the community-based research cross-cutting group were responsible for coordinating the distribution of the principles, and for facilitating linkages among interested researchers and community groups. For example, the project coordinator in Genesee County worked closely with project staff at the School of Public Health to foster community/research linkages, and to create an ad hoc subcommittee of community members to review research proposals.

Within the School of Public Health team, faculty representatives from each of the departments agreed to distribute the research principles at their departmental faculty meetings and to discuss the principles with their colleagues. To aid in this process, and at the request of team members, information was added to describe the communities and community-based organizations involved with the CBPH project, and some reasons were provided for why faculty might want to consider developing research projects using these principles and procedures. Schoolwide dissemination of the principles began in the spring of 1994, and continued throughout the following academic year.

A schoolwide forum on community-based research was held in the spring of 1995 to inform researchers at the School of Public Health about the community-based research principles and procedures, and to encourage faculty to consider conducting this type of research. The forum included presentations by faculty who had developed and implemented research projects using the community-based research principles, and information about governmental and foundation funding sources that specify community involvement in research. Thirty-five faculty, staff, and students from the School of Public Health, the School of Nursing, and the School of Social Work at the University of Michigan attended the forum.

The community-based research principles were also distributed more widely. An early version of the principles was distributed at the first CBPH Network Meeting, held in July of 1992 and attended by representatives from each of the seven CBPH consortia. The final version was also requested by, and sent to, participants from the other consortia in the CBPH Initiative. In the fall of 1994, the CBPH principles were listed in the November/December edition of the *Poverty and Race Newsletter,* distributed nationally (Poverty and Race Research Action Council, 1994, p. 15). Following the listing in that newsletter, the CBPH office at the School of Public Health responded to numerous requests for copies of the principles from community-based organizations, public health organizations, and academic institutions.

# Figure 1: Community-Based Public Health Research Principles

1. Community-based research projects need to be consistent with the overall objectives of the CBPH Initiative. These objectives include an emphasis on the local relevance of public health problems and an examination of the social, economic, and cultural conditions that influence health status and the ways in which these affect lifestyle, behavior, and community decision making.

2. The purpose of community-based research projects is to enhance knowledge and promote change in ways that benefit the community.

3. Community-based research projects are designed in ways that enhance the capacity of the community-based participants in the process.

4. Representatives of community-based organizations, public health agencies, and educational institutions are involved as appropriate in all major phases of the research process, e.g., defining the problem, gathering data, using the results, sharing and disseminating the results.

5. Community-based research is conducted in a way that strengthens collaboration among community-based organizations, public health agencies, and educational institutions.

6. Community-based research projects produce and disseminate the findings to community members in clear language respectful to the community and in ways which will be useful for community action.

7. Community-based research projects are conducted according to the norms of partnership: mutual respect; recognition of the knowledge, expertise, and resource capacities of the participants in the process; and open communication.

8. Community-based research projects follow the policies set forth by the sponsoring organization regarding ownership of the data and output of the research (policies to be shared with participants in advance). Any publications resulting from the research will acknowledge the contribution of participants, who will be consulted prior to submission of materials and, as appropriate, will be invited to collaborate as coauthors. In addition, following the rules of confidentiality of data and the procedures referred to below (Item #9), participants will jointly agree on who has access to the research data and where the data will be physically located.

9. Community-based research projects adhere to the human subjects review process standards and procedures as set forth by the sponsoring organization. For example, for the University of Michigan these procedures are found in the Report of the National Commission for the Protection of Human Subjects of Biomedical and Behavioral Research, entitled "Ethical Principles and Principles for the Protection of Human Subjects of Research" (The "Belmont Report").

# Barriers and Challenges to the Development and Early Implementation of Community-Based Research Principles

In this section we explore barriers and challenges encountered in the development and early implementation of the community-based research principles. Several of these barriers are common to community members and researchers in the process of developing collaborative projects, while other challenges are of more concern for researchers who are based in academic settings. Not surprisingly, many of these challenges are similar to the concerns raised by participants during the adoption phase of this process. To illustrate our points, we use examples from a community-based research partnership examining concerns about lead in an urban community that was part of the Detroit-Genesee County CBPH project.

**Clarification of Community-Based Research.** One challenge involved articulating clearly the vision of community-based research underlying the principles, and communicating that vision to community members and researchers from a variety of disciplines. As noted earlier in this paper, even within the group of faculty researchers who had worked most closely with this project, there were various definitions of community-based research. Therefore, communication about community-based research needed to distinguish between community-based research that emphasizes community/research partnerships and models which do not (see Hatch et al., 1993, as described earlier in this chapter). Part of the challenge was to develop a common language with which to talk about research and community concerns. Participants grappled with articulating the relevance of the principles to research conducted from a variety of disciplinary perspectives, addressing a variety of questions, and using a variety of methods.

**Communicating the Value of the Community-Based Research Principles.** A second challenge for the committee and others committed to facilitating community-based approaches to research was to communicate to potential users a sense of what might be gained by developing proposals using the process outlined in the principles. Some School of Public Health team members noted during the early discussion of the principles that researchers might find them overly prescriptive and prefer to follow more conventional research practices which were more familiar both to the researcher and to potential funders. Furthermore, as discussed earlier, there was concern among some researchers that these principles would be perceived as narrowing researchers' options and ability to determine how their research might be carried out most effectively. Once again, it was essential to communicate that these principles were intended as a guide for researchers who wished to work with community groups to integrate their research with efforts to modify the conditions that affected the community's health.

For community members, concerns regarding the principles were somewhat different. For example, when they were introduced in one community team, participants talked about their history with research which offered few opportunities for participation or influence in the research process, and few opportunities to benefit from the results. They raised questions about the extent to which community members would have opportunities to influence the research questions and be able to use the results, and the extent to which their interests would be served even if this process was followed in developing the research.

In contrast, when the principles were brought to the other community team, they were approved with relatively little discussion. However, when the first potential community-based research project – to examine blood lead levels in this urban population – was presented to this team, considerable discussion

ensued regarding the implementation of the principles. One of the community-based organizations had been working with a local activist group to protest the siting of an incinerator in the community, and saw this research as important to their efforts. They spoke strongly in support of the research as it was initially proposed (i.e., as developed by the researcher without community input). A second member of the team, who was based in an academic institution, urged the team to use the process outlined in the community-based research principles to construct a research proposal that would both meet the objectives of the researcher and involve community members.

This suggestion, which involved slowing down the application process and perhaps missing the initial deadline for submitting the proposal, was perceived by the community member as interfering with, or blocking, the conduct of the research that she believed would benefit the community. After some discussion, this issue was resolved, but it suggests that community members as well as researchers may not immediately perceive benefits in following the community-based research principles and in some instances may perceive them as slowing down or interfering with moving the research forward.

**Research Relationships Take Time, Energy, and Commitment.** Developing and maintaining community/research partnerships requires investments of time, energy, and commitment on the part of both researchers and community participants. Each partner has constraints on time and energy, and investments in community/research partnerships need to be made up front, before it is clear whether the relationship will turn into a mutually beneficial partnership.

Community-based organizations often operate with a very small budget and have enormous commitments within their communities. The time invested in a research partnership is time away from activities which may be more immediately and visibly associated with their goals and their survival. Similarly, faculty must juggle many obligations and commitments including teaching, research, publishing, administration, and community and professional service. Of these, research and publications are often more highly rewarded within the university, and faculty who do not bring in sufficient research funds and publish results may not be granted tenure or promotion. Therefore, faculty expressed concern over commitment to research projects that require high initial investments of time and energy and which may be risky in terms of the likelihood of becoming a funded, publishable research project.

In the example cited above, of research on blood lead levels, the initial proposal developed by the researcher was submitted and was not funded. Among the reasons given by the funding agency was insufficient evidence of community participation in the development of the proposal. Subsequently, the researcher worked with the Community-Academic Liaison Coordinator, a CBPH staff member with the School of Public Health, to strengthen the relationship with the community group. Subsequently, jointly developed research proposals have been submitted and funded.

**Negotiating Unfamiliar Terrain.** Both community members and researchers, working in partnership, call on skills and resources that are not always part of their existing repertoires. Researchers who are adept when communicating with other researchers about research questions, design, methods, and analysis may find it necessary to develop a new set of skills and language when communicating with community members. Community members working with researchers face challenges related to understanding research proposals that include technical language and concepts. Developing skills related to thinking about research and its potential uses are part of the process as community members become engaged in the research process. Similarly, researchers develop new skills or strengthen existing ones related to the integration of research with community intervention or action processes, or the translation of research questions, methods, or findings into information that is relevant and useful to community members.

Finally, negotiation skills were essential as community members and researchers brought together potentially very different agendas or interests. The ability to confront and address conflicts in a constructive manner and to hone skills and competencies working across differences of socioeconomic status, racial/ethnic background, or education were important to addressing these challenges. For example, again drawing upon the lead research project, in an effort to meet the deadline for the initial proposal and to establish community involvement, the researcher included the name of a community member as a coinvestigator on an early proposal. This followed a conversation with the community member, but was done without her knowledge or permission. When she learned about it, she confronted the researcher and expressed her displeasure with the use of her name on a document that she had not participated in developing. The researcher apologized and they were able to discuss and resolve the

issue. Since that time, they have worked together effectively with other community members to develop and submit subsequent proposals.

**Community-Based Research and "Good" Research.** Some researchers in particular expressed concern during the development of the principles that the integrity of research questions or tools might be compromised by involving those who are not trained in research. For example, a participant in the community-based research forum in March 1995 expressed concern about the potential for conflict between academic or disciplinary standards for research and the concerns of the community. In the discussion that followed, a second senior faculty participant noted that, in his experience, there was no necessary conflict between conducting "good" research and working collaboratively with community members. Rather, he pointed to the value of talking with community members about their experiences, concerns, and theories about the health issues that they confront, noting, "Some of my best research ideas have come from talking with people in the community."

Hatch and his colleagues (1993) discuss this issue in some detail, noting that "community involvement in, if not control over, the research process could be viewed by scientists as potentially threatening to the neutrality of science" (p. 30). They note that, despite arguments to the contrary, the idea that knowledge can be value free, that there is one objective "truth," continues to "dominate the ideology, if not the practice, of scientific research" (p. 30). As discussed earlier, the "objectivity" of science has been critiqued on a variety of counts, and the limits of more traditional forms of research have been explored (see for example, Susser, 1995; Harding, 1991). However, communicating the potential advantages of participatory community-based approaches to research, including the insights and multiple perspectives of community members who can provide a more complete understanding of complex community situations, remains an ongoing challenge.

**Conducting Interdisciplinary Research.** Community-based research, particularly intervention research, may also be interdisciplinary, bringing together researchers from multiple or diverse disciplines to address a common problem. Interdisciplinary research projects have particular challenges. They are often challenging and time consuming to pull together, requiring collaboration and negotiation among researchers from different disciplines, as well as between researchers and community

63

members. Structures and systems within academic institutions can act as barriers or disincentives to interdisciplinary research, even when researchers are committed to conducting such team efforts. For example, faculty may receive little or no credit for being listed as a "co-principal investigator" on research projects for purposes of tenure and merit review, despite investing considerable time and expertise in the conduct of the research. Disciplinary perspectives and languages differ, and researchers may need to create common understandings and languages to work together. Pulling together an interdisciplinary team of researchers and community members to develop a community-based research proposal that meets grant deadlines can be a real challenge.

**Reward Systems in Academic Institutions.** We found that researchers based in academic settings face particular challenges associated with implementing community-based research. In addition to the time invested in developing and maintaining community-based research projects, they may evolve over longer time periods and bear research results more slowly than some other types of research. Current reward structures for faculty research emphasize a strong publication record. In this system, researchers who engage in community-based research may be less likely to become tenured, to be rewarded through annual merit reviews, and may be more likely to become marginalized within their departments as a result of their choice to work within community research partnerships (see also Zúñiga, 1992). Finally, one aspect of the reward system for university faculty is the ability to bring in research grant funding. Foundations are an important source of support for community-based research projects. However, in contrast to federal funding agencies, they may not pay overhead costs; hence, academic institutions may value these grants less than those which pay overhead costs.

# Lessons Learned in the Process of Developing the Principles and Their Early Implementation

In the preceding section we identified challenges and barriers that community members and academic researchers encountered in the early phases of implementing community-based research projects. The extent to which these tensions are present is related to historical and contemporary relationships between the particular community and research institution involved, the priorities of the research institution and

its willingness to support community-based research, and opportunities to develop longstanding partnerships to address common goals. In this section, we reflect on some lessons learned about addressing these barriers in the process of developing and beginning to implement these community-based research principles.

*Build working relationships, common goals, and mutual trust.* These research principles were developed within the context of a project designed to build stronger relationships among members of vulnerable communities, health departments, and academic public health institutions. The principles and procedures developed out of the relationships that had been built among the partners, and these relationships were strengthened as we negotiated an agreement on the form and content of the research principles. Trust was established as community members and academic partners worked together on specific action projects identified by and based in the community. This history of collaboration, the development of mutual trust, and shared goals were essential aspects of the development and implementation of the community-based research principles.

The process both reflected and modeled the process that the research principles were designed to facilitate – one of collaboration, negotiation, and mutual respect. It contributed to an environment of mutual trust and accountability for the development, implementation, and application of research results within the involved community. This is particularly essential, given evidence that community and provider mistrust of research is a major barrier that must be overcome in conducting research that is integrated with action (Singer, 1993; Gamble, 1993). Even when research, practice, and community partners share a common goal, they may perceive different pathways or priorities for moving toward that goal. Willingness on the part of each partner to invest in and contribute to the agenda of the others is an essential aspect of mutual commitment.

Throughout this process, the importance of community members and practice and research partners listening to and seeking to understand each other's perspective was reinforced. Furthermore, willingness to forge compromises in which each contributes and is accountable to the other, and to apologize for infractions or mistakes made, are essential skills. Because of the power differentials inherent in the relationships between researchers and community members, and because researchers often do not live in, or experience the consequences of their actions within the communities involved, there is particular responsibility on the part of researchers to be responsive to community concerns.

*Involve diverse parties in the conceptualization and adoption of the principles.* It was essential to involve participants from diverse positions in the conceptualization and adoption of the principles. Bringing together participants representing a wide range of perspectives and engaging in a collaborative process in which, as one community member noted, "community members were around the table, not just at the table," ensured that these were integrated into the principles. The involvement of diverse groups also recognized that each partner was essential to the process of developing community-based research. Partners based in community organizations can help researchers link with interested groups and organizations to develop collaborative research projects, facilitating the development of relationships among researchers and community members. Group members who have an understanding of communities as well as the demands, limits, and potential of research can facilitate the development of common language, and common and reasonable expectations.

Finally, this process helped to develop a sense of mutual commitment and accountability, so that all partners were invested in the final product and willing to work together to ensure the best possible outcome. The development of research principles by a group of researchers or practitioners without the involvement of community members, even with the best of intentions, would be unlikely to succeed if the community members with whom they sought to work were not interested and invested in the implementation of the principles.

*Develop a common language across participants.* A part of the process of developing the community-based research principles was one of coming to a common language for talking about research and knowledge. In part, this reflects the different realities, priorities, and social positions of professional researchers, practitioners, and community members: each has access to and values different sources and types of knowledge. In addition, participants may use the same word but with different meanings, or use different language when they mean the same thing (e.g., the discussions around "ownership" described earlier).

*Recognize that the process is central to developing principles.* These principles were developed and adopted through a process of ongoing dialogue, feedback, and negotiation that occurred over the better part of a year.

In that process, participants based within universities, health departments, and community-based organizations began to develop a common language and a common understanding of each other's experiences, motivations, and perspectives related to community research. This dialogue was essential to develop mutual trust, understanding, and commitment to the implementation of the principles. Thus, we believe that these principles cannot simply be transported into a new context and adopted; the process through which they are developed is of central importance (for further discussion of the development of relationships between researchers, practitioners, and community participants, see Israel, Schurman, and Hugentobler, 1992).

*Support community members, faculty, and students involved in the process.* The CBPH project staff at the School of Public Health worked closely with faculty, public health practice professionals, and community members to develop relationships and facilitate communication that enabled them to design community-based research acceptable to all parties. Recognition that community-research partnerships involve skills, processes, and constraints that may be new to either researchers or community groups suggests the need for ongoing support, backup, and training for both research and community partners. Developing the skills and language to ask questions of researchers about their proposals – and to articulate a research project that meets the objectives of both community members and researchers – involves time and opportunities to talk with trusted others in this process. Training opportunities that highlight both potential challenges and opportunities, such as the community-based research forum, are important for facilitating community-based research. Working with a trusted third party who can help create and maintain linkages among community members and researchers, problem solve, and negotiate conflicts when they arise is another valuable strategy. At the School of Public Health, the community academic liaison coordinator – an individual with strong linkages both within the School and the involved communities – played this role.

*Acknowledge that the dissemination and implementation processes are as important as development and adoption.* Time dedicated to the dissemination and implementation of the community-based research principles proved to be as important as the development and adoption of the principles themselves. Faculty, practitioners, and community members

65

involved with the project worked together following the adoption of the principles to disseminate and interpret them throughout the School of Public Health and within the involved communities. It was through the process of implementing the principles that community members, researchers, and public health professionals began to understand more fully the implications, challenges, and steps necessary to realize the benefits of working together to develop community/researcher partnerships. For example, in designing the lead exposure study described earlier in this paper, community members supported a traditional research design that they felt would produce results that would be useful to them. In addition, they provided insights that contributed to a better understanding of the history and politics within that community relevant to the question of blood lead levels (see Hatch et al., 1993, for another discussion of the benefits of community participation).

## Implications for Community Practice and Research

In this paper we have examined the theoretical and conceptual basis for research partnerships among community members, public health practice professionals, and researchers. Community/researcher partnerships are grounded in social science perspectives that seek to link knowledge with practice. Research that engages community members as active participants may both result in more comprehensive understandings of social phenomena and establish pathways that facilitate the use of that knowledge by participants to create change within their communities. The development of such community/research partnerships, however, poses challenges for all involved.

The barriers, challenges, and lessons learned have implications for community members and researchers involved in linking research with practice. They emphasize the importance of developing long-term collaborative relationships, grounded in common goals and mutual trust, among researchers, practitioners, and members of the community. Such relationships require investments of time, energy, and funds. Academic institutions can facilitate the development of such partnerships by ensuring that faculty, practitioners, and community members are adequately supported for the additional investments required for community/research partnerships. Structural changes to support the process may include modifications in the tenure and merit review systems for faculty members, additional administrative and clerical support for community practice ventures,

and the provision of concrete support for community members and practitioners involved with the project (e.g., recognition of time invested as consultants or advisory board members, reimbursement for travel costs).

Our experience suggests that researchers, practitioners, and community members all benefit from opportunities to reflect and work through questions and concerns about the development of community-research partnerships. Information, training, and opportunities to learn through dialogue and exchange with other more experienced participants may be required for all involved. As noted above, community members, practitioners, and researchers find themselves negotiating in new and different contexts, in which communication and norms of interpersonal interactions may be a challenge: in effect, working "across cultures." Community members and practitioners may benefit from an introduction to technical terminology and basic principles of research. Researchers may benefit from an orientation to the community of concern, opportunities to develop ways of talking about technical issues in nontechnical language, and training in working across educational, racial/ethnic, and economic differences. Community practitioners may play an important mediating role between research culture and the community.

Furthermore, institutions or coalitions with an interest in supporting community-based work may create mechanisms to provide ongoing support to community-research partnerships. Such support might involve identifying potential partnerships; facilitating the development of skills for entering the field, establishing productive relationships, and communicating effectively; and anticipating or interpreting differences or conflicts. Here again, community practitioners based in community settings may play a critical role, helping to anticipate challenges and providing resources to address them.

Our experience suggests that even those faculty with the belief that a participatory community-based approach to research is appropriate and relevant to their work may find the process daunting, given the pressures of academic institutions on faculty (particularly nontenured faculty) to publish and obtain grant money. Tenured faculty may play an important role in influencing institutional merit, promotion, and tenure review policies to be more supportive of faculty engagement in carefully conducted participatory community-based research efforts.

Adherence to community-based research principles, such as those described here, can foster the development of community-research partnerships, contribute to a more complete understanding of community issues, and establish pathways that facilitate community members' use of that knowledge to address those issues. Such partnerships do not arise overnight or in a vacuum. They require time and support, from the individuals and institutions involved, and from communities and funding sources. Community practitioners, researchers, and community members all have important roles to play in this process, as well as different challenges, and resources to contribute. The investment required to develop collaborative working relationships that can translate between community practice and research has long-term benefits: it strengthens the capacity of partners to address social inequities that affect the health and well-being of the communities involved.

# References

Alinsky S. *Rules for Radicals*. New York: Vintage Books; 1971.

Austin MJ and Betten N. Rural organizing and the agricultural extension service. In N Betten and MJ Austin (eds.) *The Roots of Community Organizing 1917-1939*. Philadelphia, PA: Temple University Press; 1990.

Bailey D. Using participatory research in community consortia development and evaluation: Lessons from the beginning of a story. *The American Sociologist*. 1992; 23(4):71-82.

Brown LD and Tandon R. Ideology and political economy in inquiry: Action research and participatory research. *Journal of Applied Behavioral Science*. 1983; 19:277-94.

Cancian FJ and Armstead C. *Participatory Research: An Introduction*. Department of Sociology, UC Irvine, CA; 1990.

Chamber E. *Applied Anthropology: A Practical Guide*. Prospect Heights, IL: Waveland Press; 1985.

Clark N and McLeroy K. Creating capacity: Establishing a health education research agenda. *Health Education Quarterly*. 1995; 22(3):270-2.

Collins PH. *Black Feminist Thought: Knowledge, Consciousness, and the Politics of Empowerment*. Boston, MA: Unwin Hyman, Inc.; 1990.

Elden M. Political efficacy at work: The connection between more autonomous forms of workplace organization and more participatory politics. *American Political Science Review*. 1981; 75:43-58.

Elden M. Client as consultant: Work reform through participative research. *National Product Review*. 1983; Spring:136-47.

Elden M. Sociotechnical systems ideas as public policy in Norway: Empowering participating through worker-managed change. *Journal of Applied Behavioral Science*. 1986; 22:239-55.

Elden M. Sharing the research work: Participative research and its role demands. In P Reason and J Rowan (eds.) *Human Inquiry: A Sourcebook of New Paradigm Research*. New York: John Wiley and Sons; 1987.

Fals-Borda O. *Knowledge and People's Power: Lessons with Peasants: Nicaragua, Mexico and Columbia*. New York: New Horizons Press; 1988.

Fay B. *Critical Social Science*. Ithaca, NY: Cornell University Press; 1987.

Feagin JR and Feagin CB. *Social Problems: A Critical Power-Conflict Perspective, Fourth Edition*. New Jersey: Prentice Hall; 1994.

Fisher EB. The COMMIT trial. Editorial. *American Journal of Public Health*. 1995; 85:159-60.

Frideres JS. *A World of Communities: Participatory Research Perspectives*. North York, Ontario: Captus Press; 1992.

Gamble VN. A legacy of distrust: African-Americans and medical research. *American Journal of Preventive Medicine*. 1993; Suppl. to 9(6):35-8.

Gutierrez L. Working with women of color: An empowerment perspective. *Social Work*. 1990; 35(2):149-53.

Habermas J. *Legitimation Crisis*. Boston, MA: Beacon Press; 1975.

Hall B. Participatory research: An approach to change. *Convergence*. 1975; 11(3):25-7.

Harding S. *Whose Science? Whose Knowledge? Thinking From Women's Lives.* Ithaca, NY: Cornell University; 1991.

Harmon M and Mayer R. Interpretive and critical theories: Organizing as social action. *Organization Theory for Public Administration.* Boston, MA: Little, Brown and Co.; 1986.

Hatch J, Moss N, Saran A, Presley-Cantrell L, Mallory C. Community research: Partnership in Black communities. *American Journal of Preventive Medicine.* 1993; Suppl. to 9(6): 27-31.

Henderson D. *Feminist Nursing Participatory Research with Black and White Women in Drug Treatment.* Unpublished doctoral dissertation. University of Michigan, Ann Arbor; 1994.

Hooks B. Educating women: A feminist agenda. *Feminist Theory: From Margin to Center.* Boston, MA: South End Press; 1984.

Hooks B. "When I was a young soldier for the revolution": Coming to voice. *Talking Back: Thinking Feminist, Thinking Black.* Boston, MA: South End Press; 1989.

Institute of Medicine. *The Future of Public Health.* Washington, DC: National Academy Press; 1988.

International Council for Adult Education. *Participatory Research for Adult Education and Literacy: Principles for Practitioners.* Toronto, Ontario: International Council for Adult Education; 1980.

Israel BA, Cummings KM, Dignan M, Heaney CA, Perales D, Simons-Morton B, Zimmerman MA. Evaluation of health education programs: Current assessment and future directions. *Health Education Quarterly.* 1995; 22(3):366-91.

Israel BA, Schurman SJ, House JS. Action research on occupational stress: Involving workers as researchers. *International Journal of Health Services.* 1989; 19:135-55.

Israel BA, Schurman SJ, Hugentobler M. Conducting action research: Relationships between organization members and researchers. *Journal of Applied Behavioral Science.* 1992; 28(1):74-101.

Jaggar A. *Feminist Politics and Human Nature.* Totowa, NJ: Rowman and Littlefield; 1988.

Jaggar A and Bordo S. *Gender/Body/Knowledge: Feminist Reconstructions of Being and Knowledge.* New Brunswick: Rutgers University; 1989.

James S. Racial differences in preterm delivery. Foreword. *American Journal of Preventive Medicine.* 1993; Suppl. to 9(6): v-vi.

Lewin K. Action research and minority problems. *Journal of Social Issues.* 1946; 2(4):7-22.

Lewis E and Ford B. The network utilization project: Incorporating traditional strengths of African-American families into group work practice. *Social Work with Groups.* 1990; 13(4):7-22.

Maguire P. *Doing Participatory Research: A Feminist Approach.* Amherst, MA: The Center for International Education, School of Education; 1990.

Marin G, Burhansstipanov L, Connell C, Gielen A, Helizer-Allen D, Lorig K, Morisky D, Tenney M, Thomas S. A research agenda for health education among underserved populations. *Health Education Quarterly.* 1995; 22(3):346-63.

Mittlemark MB, Hunt HK, Heath GW, Schmid TL. Realistic outcomes: Lessons from community-based research and demonstration programs for the prevention of cardiovascular disease. *Journal of Public Health Policy.* 1993; 14(4):437-62.

Mulling L. *Race, Class and Gender: Representations and Reality.* Memphis, TN: Center for Research on Women, Memphis State University; 1992.

Paul B. *Health, Culture and Community.* New York: Russell Sage Foundation; 1995.

Poverty and Race Research Action Council. *Poverty and Race Newsletter.* 1994; 3(6).

Rogers E and Shoemaker F. *Communication and Innovations: A Cross-Cultural Approach.* New York: Free Press; 1971.

Singer M. Knowledge for use: Anthropology and community-centered substance abuse research. *Social Science and Medicine.* 1993; 37(1):15-25.

68

Smith D. *The Everyday World as Problematic: A Feminist Sociology*. Boston, MA: Northeastern University Press; 1987.

Steckler A, Allegrante JP, Altman D, Brown R, Burdine J, Goodman RM, Jorgensen C. Health education intervention strategies: Recommendations for future research. *Health Education Quarterly*. 1995; 22(3):307-28.

Steckler A, Dawson L, Israel BA, Eng E. Community health development: An overview of the works of Guy W. Steuart. *Health Education Quarterly*. 1993; Suppl. 1:S5-S27.

Steuart GW. Scientist and professional: The relations between research and action. *Health Education Monographs*. 1969; 29:1-10.

Steuart GW. The people: Motivation, education and action. *Bulletin Academy of Medicine*. 1975; 51:174-85.

Steuart GW and Kark SL. A practice of social medicine: A South African team's experiences in different African communities. *Health Education Quarterly*. 1993; Suppl. 1:S29-S47.

Stinn L. *Participatory Research: Theory and Practice*. Unpublished paper. University of Michigan, Ann Arbor; 1980.

Stoeker R and Beckwith D. Advancing Toledo's neighborhood movement through participatory action research: Integrating activist and academic approaches. *Clinical Sociology Review*. 1992; 10:198-213.

Stoeker R and Bonacich E. Why participatory research? Guest editors' introduction. *The American Sociologist*. 1992; 23(4):5-14.

Susser M. The tribulations of trials - Intervention in communities. Editorial. *American Journal of Public Health*. 1995; 85(2):156-8.

Vega WA. Theoretical and pragmatic implications of cultural diversity for community research. *American Journal of Community Psychology*. 1992; 20(3):375-91.

W.K. Kellogg Foundation. *Community-Based Public Health Initiative*. Battle Creek, MI; 1992.

Yeich S and Levine R. Participatory research's contribution to a conceptualization of empowerment. *Journal of Applied Social Psychology*. 1992; 22(24):1894-1908.

Zúñiga X. Sanctions and rewards. *Views and Issues in Action Research*. Unpublished doctoral dissertation. University of Michigan, Ann Arbor; 1992.

70

*Editors' Note: Local public health agency partners were a critical link for the Community-Based Public Health Initiative. In this chapter, the director of one CBPH consortium public health department reviews the traditional approaches of local public health, relates the strides made through the consortium's collective work, and reflects on the challenges and gains incumbent in this model. The analysis and insight based on one health department's efforts through the CBPH Initiative suggest avenues for other public agencies committed to serving communities.*

**Chapter VII** | # Community-Based Practice in Public Health

*Robert M. Pestronk*

## Public Health Agency Roles and Challenges

People who work in and govern local governmental public health agencies (henceforth, "agencies") can play a unique and important role in their communities. They specifically can do a great deal to help improve the health of the communities in which they live and serve. Personal growth, personal change, and personal leadership are required of agency staff if this is to happen.

The roles for agencies can be summarized in three areas:

1. *Assess* on a regular basis whether certain elements, essential services, processes, and outcomes are present in their jurisdiction;

2. *Develop a health policy framework* of incentives, expectations, outcomes, values, rewards, and penalties for organizations and individuals in their jurisdiction; and

3. *Assure* that health status and quality of life meet the expectations of community members, collectively, through processes which include participation, negotiation, regulation, oversight, direct service delivery, social marketing, other marketing, and strategic choice.

The resources of agencies are limited; boards of directors must choose carefully how to invest them. Strategic choice is therefore important to determine which of the many areas of possible work should be performed by, or through, the public health agency.

Opportunities to improve the public's health are increasing. Today there is a renewed interest in health and the role that each person, and people collectively, can play in becoming healthier. New partners are seeking each other out. Some have resources and guidance to share; others are looking for assistance. Local agencies, like other nongovernmental partners, bring both value and a unique perspective to efforts to improve the public's health.

Agency leaders face several challenges. One is to inform people outside the discipline about public health issues and work with their organizational leaders to achieve this goal. New partners must be welcome at the agency's table, just as agencies would be open to invitations to join other groups. In some cases, personal or professional perspectives of agency leaders must be reframed if others are to see and understand the agency's role. In still other cases, the personal and professional vision of agency leaders will need to be revised or translated into a language that is accessible to others.

A second challenge is to reshape the perspectives of those who work within our organizations and to be certain each agency's staff and associates have the requisite attitudes, skills, and knowledge to assess health status, develop community policy, and deliver services. Staff members also need to know how to facilitate community processes if they are to be responsive to individuals in local neighborhoods, and at the same time be able to assure the health of the entire community.

A third challenge is to examine the relationships between the local agency and other organizations in the same jurisdiction. Traditional and long-standing interactions must be carefully reevaluated. Current investments of energy, time, and resources must be considered against what might be possible from investing these same resources in new ways and for different purposes.

Finally, and perhaps most important, leaders must manage the process which defines the relationship between the agency itself and the residents who live in its service area. If constituents are left uninformed and remain inactive in shaping their own health – and in developing high expectations for the public health agencies that are there to protect and serve them – then all else will likely fail. Under such circumstances no community can be healthy, the public's health cannot be assured, the agency's job is incomplete, and advocacy for health improvement is left unsupported.

Local public health agencies are part of the present "system" in the eyes of many community residents. If that system were working for the health of all, communities would be healthier than they are. Indeed, if healthier communities are really the goal, some things will have to be done differently. Public health leaders will need to change, and they will need to help others do so.

Doing things differently is not easy. Friends are lost. There is conflict. New skills must be learned and practiced. Others' experiences must be considered, and possibly adopted. No two communities or health departments are identical, just as people and resources are different. Cultures also are different. There is no handbook to outline the steps for success. Nonetheless, this work *can* be done!

## Community-Based Practice

This is a practice model that can be adapted for use in any jurisdiction. It requires a change in mindset and a change from common approaches. "Community-based" means derived from the residents of a neighborhood or locale. "Practice" describes the process or methodology of the agency's work. Community-based practice is an approach that is derived from local residents.

Community-based practice rests on 10 principles:

1. Assets are foundation stones.
2. Listen first.
3. Think long-term to build trust.
4. Pay attention to *process* before product.
5. Start with the other's agenda.
6. Adopt partnerships in problem solving.
7. Expect accountability in others.
8. Be accountable.
9. Share culture and values.
10. Model by example from the top of the organization.

> *If constituents are left uninformed and remain inactive in shaping their own health — then all else will likely fail.*

*Assets are foundation stones*. Start first with what exists in the community, as described by McKnight in Chapter II in this volume and related sources (Kretzman and McKnight, 1993). Many committed individuals and organizations already are working to improve health and the quality of life in targeted neighborhoods. Seek them out through an assessment process before starting anything *de novo*.

*Listen first*. If others have the opportunity to inform your agency, listen. A window is then open for a fresh breeze to blow in both directions. Entertain the notion that those who are living with "problems" are capable, intelligent people with skills and ideas of their own. Given the scope of their challenges, their survival life skills may be better than the skills of many others. Residents and neighborhoods viewed as problematic or at "high risk" should not be discounted simply because they lack financial resources and professional know-how. There are other resources just as important and other forms of currency of value in communities. A combination of resources offers a chance to improve the public's health.

*Think long-term to build trust.* Nothing lasting or important is created overnight. Failure and frustration can precede small increments of success. Each person carries baggage from the past that can make it difficult to begin something new. What seems new to an individual may actually appear to others a thing that has been tried before. Keep in mind that many potential partners don't believe the past was all that great. Time is necessary to erode bad memories and build new foundations. Trust is the result of cumulative experience only built over time. Persevering through failure as well as success takes time and builds trust.

*Pay attention to process before product.* Consider the setting, tone, and content of personal interaction before discussion about the desired result. This can help create a climate that is supportive of change, one that helps build rules and expectations for future interactions. It can take the edge off otherwise difficult meetings and lay the groundwork for future relationships.

*Start with the other's agenda.* Offer time, financial support, or other resources to help develop another organization's agenda before starting your own. Community residents are all too familiar with short-term grant programs that are based on someone else's priorities, and that have too little relevance and too little funding (or time) to take root. Offering assistance for their priorities is a statement of your agency's respect and confidence.

***Adopt partnerships in problem solving.*** Each person or institution is endowed with assets and liabilities. Partnerships allow the liabilities of any one partner to be overcome with the assets which others bring.

***Expect accountability in others.*** Require those who use your resources to use them responsibly. It may be necessary to provide mentoring and training to assure that this occurs. But demanding high standards, requiring accurate records, and having regular reporting on what has been accomplished are part of a strong foundation. Nothing sours a good relationship faster than the inability of either party to bear public scrutiny.

***Be accountable.*** Expect from yourself and your agency staff what you expect from others outside the organization. Deliver what has been promised.

***Share culture and values.*** Be open about your agency's current organizational culture. Talk about its strengths and failings. Expect others to be equally frank. Be prepared to offer technical assistance over time to help partners better understand your agency's operating values. Be open to others who may be better informed or better prepared. It may not be possible to change bad habits and addictions quickly, and situations often look better than they actually are. It is best that partners have a realistic picture of the agency's working environment and vice versa.

***Model by example from the top of the organization.*** Staff members within any organization and members of community-based organizations (CBOs) closely observe the priorities and practice of the organization's leader to see whether the action matches the rhetoric. Organizational transformation requires leadership from the top. Since CBOs may have had negative experiences with governmental organizations (including public health agencies) in the past, personal time and commitment of top leaders is especially important if new partnerships are to be created.

# A Context for Community-Based Public Health

Community-based public health is one form of community-based practice. It is consistent with the vision spelled out in the Institute of Medicine's *Future of Public Health* (1988).

> *The committee recommends that each public health agency involve key policy makers and the general public in determining a set of high-priority personal and community-wide health services that governments will guarantee to every member of the community.* (p. 142)

> *The committee recommends the following functions for local public health units: ... policy development and leadership that foster local involvement and a sense of ownership, that emphasize local needs, and that advocate equitable distribution of public resources and complementary private activities commensurate with community needs.* (p. 145)

The context for local agency involvement in community-based public health is also described in *Blueprint for a Healthy Community: A Guide for Local Health Departments* (National Association of County and City Health Officials, 1994). This document identifies ten essential elements to protect and improve the health of communities. As listed in the *Blueprint*, they are:

- Conducting community diagnosis.
- Preventing and controlling epidemics.
- Providing a safe and healthy environment.
- Measuring performance, effectiveness, and outcomes of health services.
- Promoting healthy lifestyles.
- Laboratory testing.
- Providing targeted outreach and forming partnerships.
- Providing personal health care services.
- Research and innovation.
- Mobilizing the community for action.

Community-based public health exemplifies the tenth element – mobilizing the community for action – by providing leadership and initiating collaboration. Facilitating community empowerment is another facet of this function. There is need to do this competently and assure that agency staff members are capable and committed to the task. As stated in the document:

*The most effective local health departments are supported in their work by the communities they serve. It is the people of any community, individually and collectively, who make daily decisions which affect the health of any community. Residents of any community who seek better health can organize themselves toward that end. Local health departments with the capacity to empower communities can assist in this effort.*

*This capacity requires the ability to listen to the voices of those in a community to understand the strengths and limitations as well as the goals and behaviors of those who live in the community. It may require the ability to prevent a "professional" perspective from being superimposed on the community. It often requires the ability to prioritize work according to the needs of those in a community and build from their strengths, rather than institutional strengths. It requires opening the health department programs and procedures to increase community involvement and input in designing and evaluating programs and policies.*

*Residents of a community must possess confidence in their ability to create the conditions in which they can be healthy. Local health departments must possess the skills which can assist residents in building that confidence and, in the process, identify the health department as a partner. (pp. 29-30)*

In addition to agencies, these same principles can be applied by any other organization in the health care system, or for that matter, by any other organization. All that is required is a commitment to community-based approaches on the part of the director, staff, and boards of the institution and, ultimately, in the minds of the communities they serve.

Local public health agencies should serve the entire community. It is through and with community members and their organizations that agencies can reach those whom they should be serving, but so frequently miss. It is by building bridges between and among people in these different community sectors that new ways of seeing the world and new forms of positive expression can be

developed. It is through these relationships that systems and policies change. And it is through such relationships that health status changes can occur in a less haphazard, more equitable fashion.

A local health department can be an asset not only in delivering good public health services, but also in the ways public health practitioners perceive themselves and contribute their professional expertise to communitywide issues within and outside the health field. These benefits can be measured through the eyes of those in the community with whom agencies develop new relationships, and can be seen in outcomes of the work they do together.

## The Community-Based Public Health Partnership

The W.K. Kellogg Foundation's Community-Based Public Health (CBPH) Initiative created consortia or partnerships among CBOs, academic centers, and local health departments. Academic centers were originally conceived as schools of public health, but other academic programs were found to be equally valuable partners, including K-12 schools, undergraduate schools, graduate schools, and health professions schools other than public health. In addition, practice organizations other than local health departments can and did utilize the same conceptual framework to frame their activities and resources.

The CBPH approach was used to change the way people and their institutions think and conduct business to improve mental, physical, and spiritual health. This model can be adapted for use in all communities. The following figure illustrates the pathways for the model.[1] The three-way partnership is illustrated by the triangle, with a partner at each point, as well as by the circle indicating the common ground among the partners.

In the model, partners develop a mission statement, work plan, and an agenda to strengthen the community in which the partnership functions, as well as

> *Local public health agencies should serve the entire community. It is through and with community members and their organizations that agencies can reach those whom they should be serving, but so frequently miss.*

---

[1] The model was developed by Connie Schmitz, cluster evaluator for the CBPH Initiative.

74

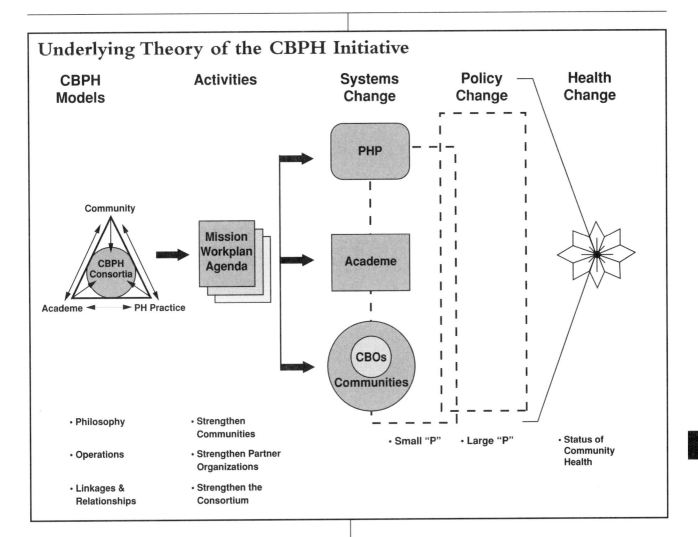

## Underlying Theory of the CBPH Initiative

CBPH Models — Activities — Systems Change — Policy Change — Health Change

Community

CBPH Consortia

Academe ◄———► PH Practice

Mission Workplan Agenda

PHP

Academe

CBOs Communities

- Philosophy
- Operations
- Linkages & Relationships

- Strengthen Communities
- Strengthen Partner Organizations
- Strengthen the Consortium

- Small "P"
- Large "P"

- Status of Community Health

the partner organizations and the consortium itself. These activities drive the *changes* needed to achieve the CBPH goals by the public health agency, the academic institution, and the CBOs. The restructuring that was needed for the agenda led to "small p" policy changes, decisions made by each participant and partner organization. As the initiative progressed over time, these changes, and the relationships and processes which formed among the partners, led to efforts to inform change in the larger umbrella under which all the partners worked. These are the "big P" policy changes made by governments, businesses, and other organizations outside the community, affecting the environment in which the community lies. Although the "big P" changes are designed to improve the health and quality of life of the general public, a side benefit is that they also improve the long-term viability of community-based partnerships.

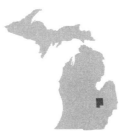

### Community-Based Public Health in Genesee County, Michigan

Genesee County is a community of approximately 430,000 people in southeastern Michigan. The department works with a budget of approximately $20 million and a staff of 165 people, divided functionally into eight main areas: the Divisions of Behavioral Health, Personal Health, Community Health, and Environmental Health, plus the Offices of Management Information Systems, Accounting, the Medical Director, and the Health Officer.

The CBPH experience in Genesee County focused initially in Flint, population approximately 140,000, located in the geographic center of the county. The project was centered in the north-central section of the city in an area surrounding the McCree Health Department building, commonly known as McCree North.[2]

---

[2] Floyd J. McCree, after whom the building was named, was the first African American mayor of the City of Flint and the first African American mayor of a large American city.

The traditional demographics and health statistics for the area surrounding McCree North indicate a predominantly African American area with high rates of unemployment, infant mortality, and chronic and communicable diseases. In 1991 it was an area in such need of safety-net services that the County Board of Commissioners was persuaded to renovate an old building as a health and human services center. The building had originally been built with Model Cities funding as a community center, with a theater, gymnasium, and offices.

Prior to the CBPH Initiative, the Health Department's outreach included print and electronic media, as well as work by internal staff to reach local residents by phone, mail, and home visits. The goal was to gather information to improve personal health and access to medical care, including health department services.

## CBPH Development and Implementation

When community leaders try to solve a problem, they usually invite each other to meet. Generally included are individuals in charge of agencies, government programs, businesses, and labor groups. Conversations evolve into a strategic planning process. This eventually leads to the development of a plan to solve or mitigate the problems of the constituents. Before the CBPH project, the Health Department's efforts had followed a similar path, either as a facilitator or a member of such groups. The approach was to be different in this instance.

Because of the concepts that emerged in preparing for the CBPH project, staff from the Health Department began to inquire about neighborhood people and issues beyond the *problems* of the McCree North area. It turned out there were some remarkable strengths that had not been known or considered.

Next to McCree North were two rather prominent buildings, an adult high school and an elementary school. None of the Health Department staff had met the people there or had been in the buildings. We decided to introduce ourselves, and to admit up front that in spite of physical proximity we had not been very helpful or active neighbors. Further, we wanted them to know that the department needed partners in its work and recognized that the schools were closer to the community in some ways than we were. We admitted that if we had known how to solve the big community health problems, the health status of the residents would be "better than it is."

This was an important recognition of the vulnerability of our agency, and an acknowledgment of the lack of success the health department and other dominant institutions in the city had had over the years in addressing the seemingly intractable problems of poverty and poor health. It was an open request for help, and a statement that the department was not approaching the community with answers, but wanted to listen and look for partners. The same approach was later used with some of the dozens of CBOs that were located in the area surrounding McCree North. These groups had been identified from a survey of neighborhood needs and assets, using methods described in Kretzman and McKnight (1993).

The Health Department subsequently selected six of these CBOs to work with as part of developing the initial CBPH proposal. Selection was on the basis that they worked actively with residents in the area immediately surrounding the McCree North building. In meetings with the six CBO directors, we hoped to listen, build trust, and begin some new relationships.

Many meetings were held over several months and these ultimately lead to the development of a proposal to the Kellogg Foundation. As part of the proposal, the Health Department committed to supporting the needs of the community from the perspective of the CBOs. It requested that each of these groups develop short proposals to describe the kinds of programs they believed would be helpful. Assistance from the department was offered where necessary to help draft the proposals. The department offered to use no grant funds to carry out its own activities should the proposal be funded.

The projects proposed by the CBOs illustrate the range of interests of these organizations and the insight that their members had in what would improve their quality of life. The proposals also reflected the aspirations of the residents and the things they would do if resources were available to finance their dreams. Not surprisingly, some requests fell outside the boundaries of the department's traditional programs. But we believed by working from *their* agenda first, the community would likely discover *public health's* agenda later.

One organization, a parent-teacher group in an elementary school, sought funding for book fairs in their school. It was their observation that most children had never had an opportunity to select a book they could call their own. Their negotiations with book companies were so successful that they produced two to three times more books per child with the funds in hand than originally had been thought possible. The leader of the organization recently recalled the first fair, and the pride on the faces of the children as they walked through the hallways carrying their books.

A second organization introduced African American male mentors into some elementary classrooms. It was the contention that most classrooms were staffed by women of European ancestry. Many children had little experience interacting with African American men, especially those who were gainfully employed.

Two organizations sought to support training programs on such topics as home renovation, plumbing, tenants' rights, and neighborhood organizing.

Another group formed a nonprofit corporation to provide transportation for child health screening appointments. The group used vans donated during the day from three local churches; the vans were returned for church use at other times. This same group also set up training programs for congregation members who wanted to help provide health care and support services.

The sixth organization hired two community members to catalogue and make known the needs and aspirations of the local residents. They encouraged local people, particularly older residents, to come out of their houses to participate in events conducted by the organization. The residents ultimately organized themselves as a block club, one that has continued to meet to address problems in the neighborhood. The proposal also requested funds for a local university to develop a catalog of career opportunities in the health and helping professions.

## Benefits of the Initiative's Community-Based, Collaborative Approach

This was the first time that many of the CBOs had talked and worked with one other. They recognized this benefit soon after the project was funded. In some cases they began to take advantage of, and recommend to others, the services and activities of their partners. Some of the joint strategies that evolved were outreach and community health worker development, nascent work in violence prevention, a challenge to a local incinerator construction project, and tenants' rights organizing.

Several of the CBOs participated in a successful local initiative to reduce tobacco use. They encouraged the County Commission to adopt regulations requiring licenses for tobacco retailers and restrictions on tobacco use in public places.

The collaboration produced some remarkably frank and refreshing discussions about race that freed participants to view each other as *people* first (Selig et al., 1993).

The CBOs and staff from the local health department joined faculty members at a local university to create and teach a course which encouraged students to adopt a community-based perspective in their analysis and understanding of local health problems (Selig and Pestronk, 1995).

A set of community-based research principles was developed by the Michigan Consortium, of which the Genesee Team was and is a part. These are beginning to be used by university faculty members as they explore research opportunities in the community. Community members bring these principles to meetings as a way of orienting investigators to a type of research that the community supports.

The Health Department learned that some of its most valuable expertise included (1) its ability to plan, budget, organize, and administer programs, and (2) its ability to write proposals which described the partnership's vision in a manner that was acceptable to funding institutions. The agency thus became a part of helping realize the community's vision. By sharing this expertise, consortium partners became interested in the other work of the department, including its data, people, and programs. Numerous orientations have been provided to the partners about the official work and programmatic resources of the agency.

Within the department we shared the experiences of the Genesee CBPH team. This process has informed and engaged staff in areas that may not have had direct exposure to project activities. This, in turn, led to several other productive relationships between CBOs, academic partners, and the Health Department. All of this has helped move the department and the community towards the mutual goal of a healthier community.

The relationships that were formed during the CBPH Initiative enhanced the value and utility of the *public health agency* in the broader community. It brought the agency to the attention of those who otherwise might have been unaware of its services. It helped reorient and improve its work. The Health

*The Health Department learned that some of its most valuable expertise included (1) its ability to plan, budget, organize, and administer programs, and (2) its ability to write proposals which described the partnership's vision.*

77

Department was able to share its experiences with the whole community, and this led other agencies and organizations to adopt a community-based approach in their own work.

For the *partner CBOs*, the project helped establish a more stable and secure base within the community with respect to funding. It engendered a growing sense of independence as their existence was validated. Other organizations started seeking them out for their own partnerships.

For the *academic* partners, there was access to productive and scholarly work with a community of residents they had not known. It meant placements for students in practice and community settings, and for community residents in academic and practice settings. It gave faculty, students, organization staff, and community residents exposure to and participation in the design and practice of community-based research.

## Generalizing the Approach for Use in Other Communities

The approach described in this chapter *can* be adapted to other settings with some thought and planning. It may require some behavior change on the part of agency personnel, however.

The CBPH Initiative was modeled with three types of organizations: local public health departments, academic institutions, and CBOs. In the Flint community, the academic organization was the University of Michigan through the Health Studies and Professions Department on its Flint campus, and the School of Public Health and the School of Social Work on the Ann Arbor campus. Conceptually, any undergraduate or graduate school with a group of faculty willing to make a commitment could be a partner. We discovered many faculty and students were eager to come forward once an opportunity was made available. It is also possible to envision public, private, or nonprofit partners other than a local health department in a community-based approach.

It is important to remember that change takes time. This can be a difficult idea to grasp in an age when we look for instant gratification. Beliefs in silver bullets and technology make us expect results quickly.

Most communities seem to be divided into two functional clusters: "experts" in institutions (the ones with the resources, degrees, etc.) and "ordinary people" in communities (those to whom services are delivered,

typically by experts in institutions). Both clusters grapple with problems of their own kind, but the world looks quite different from within each of the two clusters.

The early work in our CBPH experience required a leadership development year in which two things began to happen. First, partners in each cluster were introduced to one another through a series of lectures, seminars, workshops, travel, and other common experiences. Each side began to recognize that the other had problems, some similar and some different. Second, and perhaps more importantly, each began to identify certain assets they possessed, recognizing in some instances for the first time that these were of a different nature than those of the other partners.

Such a leadership development period is critical to success. It removes people from their own settings and introduces them to new people, different perspectives, and unaccustomed locations. As the partnership begins in earnest, bridges are built through interpersonal relationships between the experts and the people without professional expertise. The assets of one partner begin to be aligned with the problems identified by another partner.

As time passes, a culture begins to develop between these formerly isolated clusters. The word *culture* is chosen for its multiple meanings: a medium in which something can grow; a pattern of meaning commonly understood by those who are members. Asset transfer continues in the form of money, time, ideas, methods, and contacts. A transformation in perception among partners allows expertise to be ascribed to each member of the partnership. There are now experts in communities as well as experts in institutions.

As the CBPH culture supports continued growth, perceptions continue to change. Experts become people and people become experts (although experts of a different type). Community expertise becomes as valuable as institutional and professional expertise. Assets become magnified, more visible, more important, and more useful.

Continued transformation leads to a sense of shared values. Assets from all partners now begin to be applied to problems jointly identified. At its most mature stage, professionals and nonprofessionals share their expertise in a place called community. With their common values but different expertise, they develop culturally relevant solutions, mutual respect for others' expertise, and mutual trust. Each of these levels of cultural progression leads to better health and quality of life. The following figure illustrates the process.

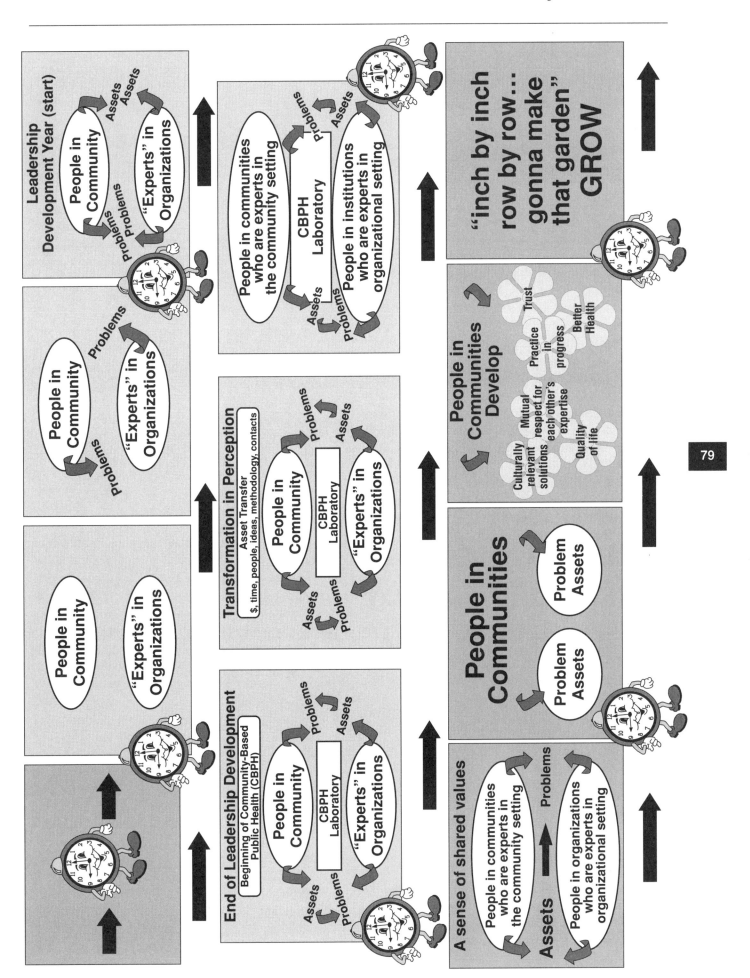

## Community-Based, Collaborative Work Continues to Enrich Community Life

Many new initiatives have developed in Genesee County out of our collective interest in and commitment to community-based practice.

In 1994, the Genesee County Board of Commissioners approved a sweeping set of tobacco control regulations which prohibits smoking in all enclosed public places, including the sports arena, shopping centers, public transport, retail stores, galleries, libraries, and centers for various types of public assembly. In addition, all retail vendors of tobacco products are required to purchase a local license to sell tobacco. Violation of the terms of the license can result in loss of the license and its privilege to sell tobacco products.

These regulations took nearly two years to pass, given the considerable controversy that surrounded them. National and state tobacco support groups flew in on many occasions to testify against the regulations. Yet a campaign to support the regulations was organized by a number of community-based groups, along with help from University of Michigan faculty and Health Department staff. Local team efforts ultimately were successful. Residents now frequently comment how pleasant it is to return to Genesee County to find public places free of tobacco smoke, after having traveled to other places.

Local youth, working under the supervision of some of our partner CBOs, have been hired to assist with regular compliance checks for those who hold tobacco licenses – part of the ongoing effort to enforce the local regulations.

Several contracts have been developed in which employees of CBOs assist the department with its work. These range from contracts to assist with outreach efforts that inform and enroll residents who are eligible for Medicaid, to campaigns to expand the numbers of ministers in the community who will support faith-based health teams in their congregations. Through our faith-based health teams, programs have been brought to audiences who might otherwise be unaware of the steps to improve health. These include tobacco cessation, healthy heart, and other chronic disease reduction activities. Contracts have been established with community organizations to conduct street corner outreach to residents at risk for (or infected with) sexually transmitted diseases, or diseases resulting from needle sharing. Local newspapers have featured the work of the "condom man" to reach a broader public.

Additional outreach and enrollment efforts are underway to reach women who may not be aware of the importance of breast examinations and Pap smears to identify cancer in early stages. These efforts provide opportunities for Genesee County residents to obtain screening, diagnosis, and treatment if they lack money or health insurance to access preventive health services.

Our faculty partners from the University of Michigan School of Public Health have begun to look to Genesee County as a site for their investigative studies. Local research efforts in the areas of cardiovascular disease, teen health, lead poisoning prevention, and cancer reduction strategies have been developed. Other community agencies have developed links with the Schools of Medicine and Dentistry at the University. We currently are exploring some joint research ventures with the National Institutes of Health and the Centers for Disease Control and Prevention.

The community-based practice model has been used as the springboard for a lead poison prevention program, in which local neighborhood and block groups identify homes that may contain high lead levels. Health Department staff join family members to give these homes a thorough cleaning, teach maintenance skills to prevent further risk, and train groups to become trainers themselves. Working with the University of Michigan School of Public Health, an interactive CD-ROM has been developed which allows students and teachers in high school and middle school to understand the nature of risk from lead. They also learn the steps that may be taken to assess, prevent, or remediate the risk. A research effort involving students and faculty has taken soil samples from throughout the city of Flint in an effort to identify the specific lead isotopes present in the community. Geographic maps will allow this information to be shared with community residents in an understandable format.

Faculty members from the University of Michigan Schools of Public Health and Medicine have initiated several other new projects that employ some of the research principles developed by the local partnerships. Partnership with the local medical society has expanded the areas of prostate cancer screening. Breast and cervical cancer research have been inaugurated through partnerships in the community, sponsored by the CBPH Consortium. We are in the process of developing new methods to reduce the rates of communicable disease, using the partnership model.

Department staff members have been gratified to see community people initiate activities independently. Support has been requested from the department and from our academic partners in a number of ways. For example, one of the earliest national court cases charging environmental racism was spawned by a group of Flint residents who opposed the location of an incinerator that burns demolition material trucked in from outside the community. Recently, these same residents stopped construction of a correctional facility in their neighborhood, proposed earlier by State of Michigan authorities.

The reason for this sensitivity to environmental health issues is not difficult to fathom. Residents already live in an area surrounded by automotive and industrial scrapyards, under the plume of the incinerator mentioned above. It is little wonder that they have organized to seek a more supportive and healthy environment.

A team comprised of representatives of the academic, practice, and community groups has been successful in obtaining funding from state and local sources to examine the local public transportation system. Hopefully, this will lead to better understanding of the ways in which that system supports access to health and human services and jobs. In this activity, as in others, students and community members are given important and meaningful roles so that those who live in the community and those who someday will be in responsible positions in other communities can draw from the Genesee partnership experiences, as well as from one another.

## Impact on Health Department Perspectives and Implications for the Future

Department staff and associates also have been stimulated by work in partnership with faculty and students. Collaborative approaches are used to introduce new skills to public health workers, and to transfer working knowledge from the field to future practitioners.

For example, efforts have been made to help all employees of the Health Department gain an understanding of the value of community-based practice. One step in this process is a series of four monthly programs open to staff department-wide. The content is based on curriculum developed by faculty and students from the University of Michigan, local community organizations, and staff from the local agency. Instructors for the training sessions are drawn from all three sources.

These sessions put teeth into a commitment to arrange regular training for department staff in areas that would enhance their work and promote the agency's strategic goals. Individual supervisors also may arrange to send their employees for training. Additionally, all staff members can request financial support to attend training programs of their own interest that may dovetail with departmental work. These efforts recognize implicitly that many of those who come to work in local health departments have neither credentials nor specific training in public health. Nor do they have training or education in the principles and values of public health practice.

A recent challenge has been to grow comfortable with the feeling of letting go, as partners become more self-sufficient and begin to develop relationships with other organizations in the community. A related challenge, one that will continue into the future, is determining the best way for existing partners to stay in touch and make use of each other as relationships with new partners develop.

Community-based practice builds on assets that already exist in the community. It strengthens and focuses resources and builds partnerships among those who already are trying to improve their quality of life and the public's health. It is an approach that can be adapted for use in many communities. Work undertaken and completed in Genesee County offers a real-life experience with this approach.

## References

Institute of Medicine. *The Future of Public Health.* Washington, DC: National Academy of Sciences Press; 1988.

Kretzman JP and McKnight JL. *Building Communities From the Inside Out.* Chicago, IL: ACTA Publications; 1993.

National Association of County and City Health Officials and the Centers for Disease Control and Prevention. *Blueprint for a Healthy Community: A Guide for Local Health Departments.* Washington, DC; 1994.

Selig S, Brown A, Brown R, Pestronk R. Using racial tensions to strengthen coalitions and promote primary care services in an economically depressed community. Paper presented at the Annual Meeting of the American Public Health Assocation; 1993.

Selig S and Pestronk R. Working toward community-based public health: The experience of Flint, Michigan. *The Link.* 1995; 7:1 and 6.

81

*Editors' Note:* This chapter details both the process and products of the CBPH Initiative's National Policy Task Force. The experiences of CBPH Initiative participants as they sought to collectively identify policies related to public health objectives, manage conflicts and perspectives among partner groups, and endorse a course of action acceptable to all consortia mirror the challenges many diverse groups face in addressing policy issues. By recounting the path CBPH consortia members took, Toby Citrin shares lessons for community coalitions, advocacy groups, and philanthropic organizations seeking to support productive changes in public health and the education of public health professionals.

| Chapter VIII | # Policy Issues in a Community-Based Approach |
|---|---|

*Toby Citrin*

The Community-Based Public Health (CBPH) Initiative not only sought to develop demonstrations of the effectiveness of community-based approaches to public health, but to inform policy discussions to support these approaches over the long term. Successful demonstration projects need to be institutionalized, expanded, and replicated if their ultimate potential is to be realized. In the case of the CBPH Initiative, if the community-based partnership approach to public health enhanced and strengthened the public health mission, that approach should be widely disseminated and related principles incorporated into policies affecting future work. As a result of dissemination efforts, discussions at the federal, state, and local government levels, as well as institutional practices and policies in health agencies, academic institutions, and community-based organizations, would reflect CBPH lessons – and ultimately the manner in which public health is taught, practiced, and funded.

This chapter defines "policy" as it was defined and addressed by the CBPH consortia. It describes policy-informing activities at the consortium level and at the national level. It identifies the barriers encountered and accomplishments achieved as CBPH partners grappled with policy implications at each level of the initiative's work. And finally, it describes the plans for expanding the CBPH model of teaching and practicing public health in the future.

## Defining "Policy" for the Community-Based Public Health Initiative

As CBPH consortia began consciously to address the policy implications of their collective work, it became evident that the term "policy" had very different meanings for each of the three kinds of CBPH partners. For academics, "policy" is a recognized academic discipline, involving the study of the processes by which institutions and organizations develop and adopt laws, rules, guidelines, and standard practices which govern their future activities. Policy studies at a university typically include political science, policy analysis, economics, and resource allocation. The "real world" activities of policy development and policy adoption are engaging not only in their own right, but because they are subjects to be studied, analyzed, and informed by research.

Public health practitioners view policy as the articulation of the rules, financing patterns, and guidelines within which they formulate and implement programs and deliver services. As seen by the authors of the 1988 Institute of Medicine's *The Future of Public Health* report, public health policy is developed by connecting knowledge developed through public health "assessment" with societal values and priorities. It is embodied in programs and services reflecting the policies adopted, thus carrying out the "assurance" function. The Institute of Medicine report sees "policy develop-

83

ment" as midway between "assessment" and "assurance" in the dynamic expressed by the linked triad of public health core functions.

For grassroots community-based organizations, the term "policy" is an abstract concept not clearly related to the quality of life of the community, even though many community residents do, in fact, engage in activities to address policy issues. While the *effects* of policy decisions often raise concerns and trigger actions in the community, the terms "policy" and "policy development" are rarely used to describe these actions. Thus, a community leader who says she has little time to get involved in policy activities may write letters, join a bus trip to the state capitol, or attend county board hearings to protest the start-up of an incinerator in the neighborhood. The CBPH Initiative cluster evaluators found that in using the terms policy and policy development in surveys and interviews of community residents, there was little interest in the activity. The same community members, on the other hand, often shared stories about the activities they undertook to change how local authorities went about their business.

The three different ways CBPH partners defined policy reflect differences in the starting points and primary concerns of each group. *Academics* view policy from the perspective of those who study and teach. Their starting point is the university, the place where research and teaching take place. They focus on places and people where the process of policymaking takes place. Their concerns are often research-oriented, represented by "academic questions" that seek to illuminate the interaction of the various forces that contribute to policymaking. They also search for the factors that make for success or failure in policy adoption and implementation.

*Public health practitioners* view policy from the perspective of their role as implementers. Their starting point is the public health department or health care organization. Their primary concerns are the rules, guidelines, and budgets of those to whom they report and those who fund their activities. They are directly affected by these policy decisions, and thus are more closely related to policy decisions than either faculty members or community residents. Consequently they are apt to express concern and interest in the policy process. But their interest is largely driven by impact on their professional practice, as distinguished from the

interest of the academic in the more abstract questions of research and teaching.

The starting point for *community residents* is the daily lives of people in the community. Their concerns are the problems encountered in earning a decent living, maintaining a clean and safe environment, and improving the quality of their own lives, that of their children, and their neighbors. Their initial focus is not on the places where policies are made but rather on the impact these policies have on their daily world. They are led into concerns about policy as the result of personal experiences, rather than their more abstract commitment to policy development. Their interest in policy is often proportionate to the geographic proximity of the actions of the governmental agency or legislative body to their homes. While academics and practitioners are inclined to look first at policymaking and then its impact on constituent groups, community residents usually reverse this process, looking first at their daily needs and then at the way these are affected by policy decisions.

The scope and timing of policymaking also differ as seen by the three CBPH groups. Academics are usually concerned about policymaking at a macro level – federal, state, and, less frequently, local and institutional policymaking. They study policymaking as it has occurred over large time spans. Practitioners are concerned about policymaking at whatever is the level of their own jurisdiction or the jurisdiction directly affecting them. They usually are willing to invest effort in policy initiatives that span budget periods or terms of office. Community residents are inclined to be most concerned about policies affecting themselves, their families and immediate communities – a particular slice of the larger policy horizon. Their efforts most often center on local government and, occasionally, state government. Community residents are likely to be skeptical of the value of time spent in policy activities that impact only long-term results. They see, instead, the many immediate tasks that need to be addressed in the daily challenges they face.

As representatives of the three CBPH partners began their series of meetings to discuss policy implications for their collective efforts, they recognized their differing perspectives on policy. They came to realize that they were equally interested, but from very differ-

> *For grassroots community-based organizations, the term "policy" is an abstract concept not clearly related to the quality of life of the community, even though many community residents do, in fact, engage in activities to address policy issues.*

ent vantage points. They hammered out a mutually acceptable definition of policy to reflect all three perspectives, incorporating not only a static definition but also the qualities which they wanted to see reflected in future policymaking:

*The Task Force has defined policy as decisions made by public, private, professional, and community groups and organizations, and by individuals, to affect behavior and to direct resources. Such decisions become "CBPH policy" when they are based on values and a process respecting the unique contributions of each of the three kinds of CBPH partners (community-based organizations; local health departments; universities), and are intended to achieve an improved quality of life.*

## Informing Policy Discussions at the Local Level

As representatives of the three CBPH partner groups continued their conversations, they shared stories about the efforts being made by CBPH consortia to disseminate what was being learned through consortia efforts and inform policy discussions in communities and institutions. They found that all CBPH partners were actively engaged in informing local policy discussions. Here are some examples:

• As the result of combined efforts of one CBPH consortium, its school of public health revised the criteria used in its merit review process by adding language on the value of community service, and it added a community faculty member in a new tenure-track position.

• One consortium brought about change in its health department's tuberculosis screening programs by training and enabling neighborhood health workers to do skin tests.

• Two consortia provided information and informed discussions related to reducing substance abuse. In one area, county ordinances tightened up control on the sale of cigarettes to minors; in another, a local community banned advertisements of alcohol and tobacco.

• One consortium shifted county funds to CBPH coalition partners to support a smoking cessation program.

• One community was faced with the impending operation of a new incinerator that threatened to increase levels of lead in the air, located in a neighborhood already experiencing elevated blood lead levels in children. Through the organized advocacy of partner organizations, and using research findings from their university partner and legal advice from the university's legal advocacy clinic, new controls were imposed on the incinerator. The permitting practices of the state environmental protection agency were changed, and court-imposed monitoring procedures were established.

• Connections fostered through one consortium made it possible for a community to address issues related to a proposed rezoning that would have allowed a highway to be built through one of its neighborhoods.

## Barriers to Community-Based Policymaking

While these and other stories suggest the potential of the CBPH approach, the attempts brought into focus some significant barriers which must be overcome if public health is to expand the scope of community-driven changes in the future. These barriers include:

• Different languages used by academics, practitioners, and community members.

• Differences in power and resources among partners, especially community members and professionals.

• The perceived difficulty of validating the work of community advocates.

• Lack of time and financial resources to support the policy-informing activities of small community-based organizations.

• Lack of trust among government, academe, and community.

• Hesitancy of university faculty and agency professionals to take the risks of putting themselves "on the line" by advocating on behalf of community interests or priorities.

• Potential loss of status among peers by identifying with the other partner groups and sharing with them in risk-taking.

• Difficulty of securing broad grassroots participation of community residents, even when the community-based organization is actively engaged.

• Lack of community ownership of the problem being addressed, often based on the suspicion of it reflecting "someone else's agenda."

85

These barriers speak to the difficulty of achieving a truly representative process in modern America and are not confined to low-income communities. Even affluent communities must work to overcome these barriers – and affluent citizens are more likely to share the language of professionals and academics, to have the time to invest in addressing policy issues, and to connect with or make contributions to advocacy groups. Affluent citizens also are more apt to be personally familiar with individuals in positions of power and influence, and to have access to support functions through their offices (secretarial support, phone, fax, and meeting space) to carry out objectives. Yet active involvement in the policy process is rare in any community. The challenges CBPH Initiative partners faced were not unique to their communities, but almost commonplace in a modern democracy.

## Overcoming the Barriers

On the positive side, the CBPH experience illustrated that the partnership approach made it possible to overcome many of these barriers. Among the opportunities and supports identified by the CBPH Policy Task Force were:

- Partnerships with universities and health agencies result in capacity building for community-based organizations.

- Combining "people power" from communities with facts and arguments generated by university and practice organizations (e.g., coupling information on environmental impacts on health with community advocacy for environmental improvement) produces credible voices for change.

- University-based evaluation of demonstration projects can support efforts to gain expanded funding for programs benefiting the community.

- Sharing funding among partners can maintain the support and involvement of fragile community-based organizations.

The challenge for community-based partnerships has been to strengthen the role of grassroots organizations by sharing skills and knowledge and building community capacity to inform the policy process. The balance of this chapter describes how the seven CBPH consortia worked together to promote the collective goal of informing policy discussions to support community-based approaches to public health.

## Building an Initiative-Wide Approach to Addressing Policy Issues

The four-year CBPH project witnessed three separate attempts to develop a national approach to informing policy discussions related to community-based public health. That the initial two attempts failed to gain the support of the seven CBPH consortia is instructive. We will consider the two failed attempts to articulate an initiative-wide approach before describing the third successful movement.

After the initial implementation year, several members of CBPH consortia urged the Kellogg Foundation to establish a committee to consider contextual policy issues that affected the work of the consortia. As a result, a committee was formed with one member chosen from each of the seven consortia. Committee members met several times and conducted a survey among the consortia to determine the nature and extent of each consortium's activities, plus the interest of each partnership in engaging in developing an initiative-wide approach to identifying policy issues.

At the 1994 Annual Network Meeting in Baltimore, Maryland, the policy committee recommended a series of actions to the combined consortia. These included the development of an initiative-wide approach for informing policy discussions at the national and state levels and the formation of a coalition to address related policy issues (including health care reform and licensure and certification related to the provision of health services).

To the surprise and dismay of committee members, the recommendations elicited reactions ranging from skepticism to opposition. CBPH participants felt that the committee was not representative of the consortia, especially the community component, that the committee was moving too fast, and that the partnerships had to build strength and cohesiveness before an initiative-wide approach could be formulated. Specifically there was a concern that community-based organizations needed to be strengthened before engaging in additional activities related to the recommendations. Members also voiced concerns that the proposed activities would be dominated by academic and practice partners. Based on the reaction of CBPH participants, the committee did no further work; the survey was filed to be available for future use.

The second attempt to formulate an initiative-wide approach to informing policy discussions was an internal activity by the W.K. Kellogg Foundation.

Foundation program staff began work on an Integrated Action Plan (IAP), a strategic planning tool that linked the activities of communication and evaluation with policy work related to initiative objectives. Once the IAP reached draft form it was shared with representatives of the seven consortia at a midyear meeting in Massachusetts – only six months after the Annual Network Meeting in Baltimore. The draft IAP brought an even stronger negative response from consortia participants than the policy committee's recommendations had. Participants expressed concerns that the Foundation's strategy was too far removed from the immediate concerns of the individual consortia and their members; that it did not reflect their collective perspectives, knowledge, and experience. Based on the response of CBPH partners, the Foundation agreed to use the IAP as an internal planning tool only.

It was now two and one-half years into the four-year CBPH project, and there was no concerted, initiative-wide effort to relate CBPH consortia efforts to a strategy that would disseminate, support, enhance, and expand CBPH work at the conclusion of the granting period. Recognizing the need to address this gap, a new Policy Task Force was convened at the end of the project's third year. The new Task Force included representation from all seven consortia and, within each consortium, of all three types of partners – 21 members plus a chair. A team from the University of Michigan and a consultant from the University of Illinois were attached to the Task Force to provide staff and logistical support.

## Managing the Process and Related Conflicts

The initial meeting of the Task Force was an attempt by the staff to plunge into the work, concentrating on achieving some initial decisions on agenda, timetable, and goals. The meeting was awkward, with little input by several of the community-based organization representatives. There was an evident lack of consensus on major issues, and a general lack of enthusiasm for the group's assigned tasks. Toward the end of the meeting, one of the community-based representatives voiced concern that the group was starting out wrong – that at least initially it needed to pay more attention to process

*The challenge for community-based partnerships has been to strengthen the role of grassroots organizations by sharing skills and knowledge and building community capacity to inform the policy process.*

than outcomes to assure that the group could come together with a shared desire to reach common goals.

The Task Force leadership and staff sharply revised the process for the next few meetings, beginning the second meeting with an "around the table" expression of why each member was there. Most of that meeting involved Task Force members sharing stories of how their organization or consortium had been working – sharing successes, failures, and valuable insights. As subsequent meetings were held, the group began to attain a better sense of shared mission. When finally the group was able to come together around a set of agreed-upon recommendations, it was clear that the initial investment of time in building mutual trust, understanding, and cohesiveness had been well worth the effort.

In the course of the Task Force's work some conflicts were never completely resolved. These issues, carried to the extreme, might have doomed the group's collective efforts. The nature of these conflicts illuminates not only historic issues, but the problems which will be encountered as the consortia seek to promote community-based policy change in future years.

First, Task Force members found that their work was perceived as an activity remote from the work of the consortia they represented. Thus, while each Task Force member was charged with the responsibility of maintaining continuous communications with his or her constituent organizations "back home," such feedback turned out to be sporadic and incomplete. Policy issues identified by the Task Force were seldom the focus of local consortium discussions and decision making. In their site visits to consortia, CBPH cluster evaluators found that the Task Force was often perceived as an activity unrelated to local work of the local consortia. This conflict between the need for the Task Force to accomplish its goals, and the desire of the Task Force to be representative of views, concerns, and interests of the constituent consortia demonstrates one of the challenges of drawing diverse partners into a common approach to informing policy discussions. One can only assume that other community-based partnerships seeking to identify and address wide-ranging policy issues will encounter similar problems. The lesson learned by the Task Force was that continuous communication between community-based groups and those who carry the responsibility for representing their interests is crucial to the success of this approach.

87

Another issue that plagued the Task Force was the traditional "process vs. outcome" conflict. Throughout the process, the Task Force had to steer a course midway between the desires of some (usually community representatives) who felt it was moving too quickly and the desires of others (usually academic or practice representatives) who felt the process was moving too slowly. The former wanted to elicit more views from each of its members and their constituent organizations, letting decisions "settle in" over time. The latter wanted to make more prompt decisions on a predetermined timetable, regardless of the extent to which some Task Force members were left out of active discussion and decision making.

The lesson learned in coping with this conflict was that if there was a sincere desire to promote community-based approaches, the group had to be willing to invest extensive time to ensure the community had a meaningful voice in the process. Professionals who are familiar with tasks related to informing policy discussions – writing documents, gathering data, articulating opinions – will always tend to dominate unless there is a conscious attempt to "slow down" and patiently elicit the views of those less experienced. The payoff at the end of the process, of course, is the solid support of decisions ultimately made by the entire group, which then translates into a strong showing of community interest.

A third persistent tension for the Task Force centered on choice of language and communication methods. Task Force members managed an ongoing conflict between the stereotyped, relatively abstract language of professionals, especially those in academe, and the more narrative language of community members. Throughout the Task Force's work, its university-based staff "translated" the output of each meeting into documents, only to find that these were seen by the consortia as overly detailed, too technical, and irrelevant to their immediate needs and concerns. As time went on, however, the Task Force and its staff came to recognize that the language of the community, often expressed in stories, was helpful in gaining the support of other communities and ultimately more powerful than the language of professionals in moving decision-making bodies to action. At the final Annual Network Meeting, when all CBPH consortia unanimously adopted the recommendations of the Task Force, a critical element in that support was not the ponderous document mailed out in advance of the meeting, but the moving stories told by community members. Those stories – illustrating how collective action can bring about meaningful change in community, and reflecting

the pride and self-esteem gained in the process – resonated in a way that no formal document could.

Another inherent conflict experienced by the Task Force was related to race. While Task Force members bonded over the 18 months of meetings, the experiences and perspectives of representatives from predominantly minority communities differed from those of many academic and agency leaders. Those differences, although not evidenced by antagonism or race-based arguments on issues, were reflected in the approaches Task Force members took on the process, and mirrored in strategy formulation and recommendations for activities.

The role race played in the Task Force's work was most strikingly evidenced at the second meeting when members broke into groups according to partner types (community-based organizations, academic institutions, and public health agencies). Virtually all African American and Latino participants represented community-based organizations. Those who reported on the dialogue among this group of community members noted the sharp differences in style and content in that discussion, compared with discussion in the larger group. This experience, duplicated in a subsequent Annual Network Meeting, led to the decision to form a separate but related organization of CBPH community partners, where participants could formulate and articulate their own objectives. The lesson learned was that minority community members and organizations need to have their own discussions – to develop their own strengths and strategies – in order to work effectively with professional partners (academics and health practitioners).

Finally, the Task Force experienced continuing conflict in the arena of setting priorities. The Task Force had an agenda centered on informing policy discussions to support long-term change; individual CBPH consortia's priorities were related to sustaining project efforts beyond the grant period. While this conflict was specific to the four-year CBPH Initiative, it mirrors a continuing polarization between the objectives of many advocacy organizations and the immediate "survival" priorities of their grassroots members.

## Task Force Accomplishments

The Task Force succeeded in accomplishing its work by balancing these conflicts as it proceeded incrementally to define "policy," to articulate a vision of community-based public health, to identify the policies which would promote that vision, and to suggest the kind of organization which might best inform those policies.

In addition to the definition of "policy" adopted, the Task Force articulated a vision of community-based public health as follows:

- The community lies at the heart of public health. We all recognize that the protection and improvement of the community's health is best achieved through the full participation of the community at the grassroots level in the selection, design, and implementation of prevention programs. Success with public health policies and programs depends upon the extent to which they reflect the community's values and priorities.

- Public health, broadly defined, embraces virtually all of the community's priorities, and provides an organizing framework for the development of programs to address them. Public health encompasses the physical, mental, social, economic, and spiritual health of the community. Public health recognizes that jobs, decent housing, the elimination of poverty, an end to racism, and economic justice are all necessary ingredients to a comprehensive health strategy.

- We believe strongly in the value of the CBPH partnership. Each of the partners (community-based organizations, local health departments, and universities) feels better able to achieve organizational objectives and to achieve our joint objectives because of having linked up with the other two partners. We all want this partnership to be strengthened, maintained, and expanded.

Next the Task Force began pursuit of related objectives: identifying both the kinds of policies that would promote the vision, and strategies best suited to informing policy discussions at the federal, state, and local governmental levels, and within health departments and universities. Additional recommendations were developed in two parts – recommendations related to informing policy discussions and organizational strategies. The seven CBPH consortia unanimously adopted both sets of recommendations at the 1996 Annual Network Meeting in Washington, D.C.

## Policies Related to Sustaining and Advancing the CBPH Approach

The Task Force identified policy issues related to the sustainability and advancement of CBPH principles at the national, state, local, and institutional levels. They included: (1) policies that would enhance the ability of community-based organizations to protect and promote

the health of citizens; (2) policies promoting partnerships between community-based organizations, health agencies (both public and private), and universities; and (3) policies advancing the vision of community-based public health. Some priority items identified included:

- Modifying academic policies to promote community-based teaching and research (e.g., changing accreditation standards and faculty incentives at public health and other health professions schools).

- Informing the policy discussions of public health agencies and health care providers to promote an effective voice for communities (e.g., roles for community-based organization leadership on boards of health; funding for training of neighborhood-based health workers; flexibility to contract with community-based organizations for carrying out components of public health programs).

- Informing state-level policy discussions related to health care organizations and the benefits they provide to communities.

## A New National Organization

The Task Force recommended the creation of a national organization which would support efforts to inform policy discussions at national, state, local, and institutional levels. A Task Force working group was charged with developing a detailed plan for the new organization, and after several months of sustained effort, the Task Force adopted the recommended plan. An initial governing board was appointed, and the W.K. Kellogg Foundation provided start-up funding.

The new organization, the Center for the Advancement of Community Based Public Health, now carries the torch lit by the CBPH Initiative. Its mission statement charges the organization with "the advancement of 'community-based public health,' i.e., the protection and improvement of community health through the full participation of the community." The Center further seeks to improve the public's health by building and maintaining local partnerships which include community-based organizations, universities, and public health agencies at the local level, and informing policy at all levels to promote community-based public health and related partnerships.

The current activities of the Center emphasize two areas: (1) providing technical assistance to organizations seeking to establish or strengthen meaningful partnerships between community-based organizations, health care providers and public health agencies, and universities; and (2) informing policy discussions to support the CBPH approach to public health.

## Conclusion

The CBPH Initiative has moved into a new era. While the original CBPH consortia have changed in organizational composition and pursuits, the vision and spirit of the initiative remain very much alive. Virtually everyone deeply engaged in the CBPH project came away from it transformed. At meeting after meeting – whether national, local consortia, or Task Force – individuals from diverse backgrounds and their organizations gave testimony to the way the project enabled them to experience the enormous potential of the CBPH partnership model.

If the CBPH vision is to be fully realized, both the practices and policies shaping public health and the education of public health professionals will need to continue to evolve. To a large extent, the CBPH vision requires a shift in power, promoting new roles in the health system for community people and community-based organizations often underrepresented in decision making. These changes will not come about because a few public health academic and practice leaders, with occasional funding from foundations, try to impose their vision on those who determine the structure of our health systems. Significant change will occur only when groups that have experienced the potential of the CBPH vision focus their collective efforts, share their experiences and skills with others, and join together to inform policy discussions related to their long-term goals. This is the dynamic set in motion by the new national organization – a dynamic characterized by Quinton Baker, the organization's executive director, as a "movement" in the way that the struggle for civil rights was a "movement."

The barriers to success, as evidenced by our experience on the Task Force, may be formidable. But the CBPH experience suggests that these barriers can be overcome, resulting in the advancement of public health's mission, and healthier communities across the United States.

*Editors' Note: Cluster evaluation of the CBPH Initiative made it possible to chart progress toward goals and begin to ascertain the overall impact of the work on participants and communities. In this review, the CBPH cluster team director summarizes information on partnerships, shared leadership, collaboration, and capacity building. She also provides analysis and recommendations for philanthropic organizations, community-based partnerships, and evaluators engaged in related public health initiatives.*

| Chapter IX | # Assessing the Community-Based Public Health Initiative: What Did We Learn? |
|---|---|

*Connie C. Schmitz*

## Introduction

Speaking for the evaluation team that traveled the distance with this initiative – from its first Leadership and Model Development meeting in Chicago in 1991 to its last annual networking conference in Washington, D. C., in 1996 – I can bear witness: The CBPH Initiative was a terrific experience in capacity building and partnership for many, many people. At last count, during the four years of implementation (1992-96), approximately 500 people from 67 organizations in 7 states were engaged. They came from schools of public health, medicine, social work, and other disciplines aligned with the health professions. They came from health departments at the state, county, and city levels. They came from community clinics and tribal governments, public schools and social action agencies; from places of worship and networks of service and advocacy. Most came with very personal commitments. Both the hope and the labor of working together to accomplish complex goals were important: the effort *meant something.* When the dust had cleared, a strong majority felt that the benefits of involvement outweighed the costs, and the clearest benefits were those relating to personal and professional growth.

As described in earlier chapters, the CBPH Initiative consisted of seven consortia, each comprised of academe, public health practice, and community partners. Each consortium was funded to "create new models of public health." This chapter will not repeat the dimensions of the initiative, but rather convey the cluster evaluation team's perspective of some of the main findings and lessons learned. We do so with the belief that the CBPH project – while unique and different in some ways – was and is similar to other large-scale, partnership-driven initiatives addressing complex societal issues in

health. As such, this chapter may be useful to others working in community-based programming.

For readers unfamiliar with the term "cluster evaluation," the concept warrants some explanation. Cluster evaluation is "evaluation of a program that has projects in multiple sites aimed at bringing about a common general change" (Sanders, 1997, p. 397). As elaborated by Sanders, in cluster programming "...projects are relatively autonomous. Each project develops its own strategy to accomplish the program goal, uses its own human and fiscal resources to carry out its plan, and has its own context" (ibid.). As summed up by the W.K. Kellogg Foundation (WKKF) director of evaluation, "Cluster evaluation is a mechanism for gathering information to use in determining the extent to which WKKF grants are helping people improve their quality of life" (Millett, 1995, p. 3).

As practiced in this instance, cluster evaluation was a systematic effort to examine, describe, and reflect on what the CBPH Initiative was about in order to help its overall progress, and then to assess the extent to which the initiative achieved its aims.

The cluster evaluation team gathered information that would help:

1. Describe the CBPH models as they were being developed across the sites;

2. Assess their effects on community capacity building;

3. Assess their effects on organizational "systems" change in academic institutions, public health agencies, and community organizations;

4. Ascertain the impact of the initiative on local or national policymaking; and

5. Document the perceived costs and benefits of participation for the individual members and organizations involved in the undertaking.

The evaluation team's work was conducted through annual site visits, conferences, and meetings; routine collection of numerous indicators relating to consortium activities/accomplishments; surveys administered to CBPH members at the end of the second and fourth years; and a video documentary. Our stance was at a medium distance: we were not *of* the projects, nor *of* the Foundation, but we worked closely *with* these stakeholders, and we shared our findings and suggestions with them as the initiative progressed.

The cluster evaluation was not "theory-based" (Weiss, 1995); it did not test hypotheses or set out to prove causal relationships through a classically designed research study. We could not, and did not, answer for all time the question, Did taking a community-based approach improve the community's health? Neither was the cluster evaluation an amalgam of seven detailed case studies. As a cluster team, we looked for themes and trends that transcended projects. Because the cluster evaluation team had interdisciplinary skills and interests, we brought an eclectic tool kit and a "user-focused" (Patton, 1997) mind-set to the task. As a result, the cluster evaluation was designed to fit the contours and nature of a developmental initiative and to respond to the interests of the primary stakeholders involved. Only individual readers can determine if our findings are generalizable to other situations.

The CBPH cluster evaluation took place during an era of intense scrutiny and interest in community-university partnerships. Because of that and the Kellogg Foundation's initial commitment to sponsor an initiative in health professions education, the evaluation team looked a bit harder at academe and the changes occurring there (e.g., in curriculum and instruction, faculty and students' experiences) than in public health practice, or in community life. Fortunately, change in the academic arena was also the most easily studied, partly because academic participants were accustomed to identifying and documenting their activities. For more detailed information on the outcomes produced by academic and other organizations, readers can request copies of the cluster evaluation team's final report (Schmitz et al., 1996).

## Overall Findings: Highlights from the Guiding Evaluation Questions

Overall, we learned that the seven CBPH consortia were very diverse in membership and structure. Not surprisingly, they identified somewhat different priorities within the common goal areas, and different strategies for addressing those goals. The following section provides an overview of what the cluster evaluation team learned vis-a-vis our five "guiding evaluation questions." These questions were generated in the CBPH Initiative's first year during meetings with consortia leaders and Foundation staff. The questions subsequently guided data collection methods.

### What kinds of collaborative, community-based public health models were developed?

- All seven CBPH consortia shared a similar theoretical orientation that embraced collaboration as a *model* of practice, and principles of community capacity building as a necessary corollary for improving public health research, education, outreach/public service, and professional practice.

- In order to accommodate the many organizations, constituencies, and people involved in multiple community sites, the organizational models that emerged tended to be quite elaborate. Most were multilevel structures, with a central governance body coordinating work across several smaller coalitions, or subgroups, operating at disparate geographic sites. According to survey data and interviews, these organizations tended to be "high maintenance" structures that required considerable skill, resources, and time to sustain. Perhaps because of this, more "success" (in terms of mutually satisfying and productive relationships) was reported at the local coalition site levels than at the central consortium level.

- The capacity to work collectively in consortia appeared to depend on many factors, including: close geographic proximity, previous positive working relationships or experiences with collaboration, strategic process skills, comfort with multicultural diversity, and a "true" impetus or basis for partnership.

- The ability of consortia to effect "systems" change and inform policy discussions (intended outcomes of the initiative) depended on the strength of the partnerships between academic, public health practice, and community members. Stronger CBPH partnerships had a high degree of member involvement and commitment from the participating organizations. They also tended to have neighborhood organizations with a history of working in the communities involved. They demonstrated high quality project direction and leadership across all three sectors (i.e., academe, public health practice, and community), and the ability to plan for and use evaluation data.

- While all consortia worked productively on some goals and activities, much of the work was in fact done by individual partner groups, working separately in parallel to each other, or together but with only one other sector. Capitalizing on the synergy of all three partnering sectors proved unrealistic for some consortia, due to geographic distance, or unproductive for others, due to lack of common goals, interests, or mutually reinforcing relationships.

- Some of the most important outcomes reported by participants were the "enduring relationships," "social networking opportunities," and "increased understanding of, and access to each others' cultures." These relationships were (for the most part) at the individual level; they depended on the chemistry of specific people. Relationships, in other words, were personally (as opposed to organizationally) contracted. Thus, the extent to which partnerships will be *institutionalized* at the organization level (irrespective of the people involved) remains to be seen.

### How did participation in the CBPH Initiative affect the community's capacity to solve public health problems?

- To answer this question, we all had to grapple with the definition of "community." Generally speaking, the process of defining community was not done systematically or consistently across the initiative. In some consortia, a "community of solution" definition was adopted. (A *community of solution* approach links individuals, groups, and organizations needed to solve an identified problem, and calls this group "the community.") More typically, however, "community" referred to those people who lived and worked in a targeted neighborhood and who experienced problems or needs that public health agencies commonly address. By this definition, institutions and agencies that serve those individuals are excluded from the meaning of community. In some consortia, the difficulty of achieving local consensus over the term "community," or the philosophy behind a true "community-based" approach, became a "cost" for the consortium in terms of conflict.

- Most community partners were involved early in CBPH, but some were recruited after the grant was awarded, and still others joined as late as the third or fourth year. The diversity of community partners (and their sense of ownership for the project) meant, among other things, that they brought very specific capacities to the project as well as varying needs for capacity building.

- The capacity building took two primary approaches: (1) increasing the capacity of community-based organizations (CBOs) and their leaders to organize and mobilize residents around public health issues, and (2) increasing the capacity of community representatives to "sit at the table" and work collaboratively with members from academe and public health practice. In some consortia, leaders recognized that these two separate kinds of capacity-building needs existed. They then found the time, money, and opportunities (both formal and informal) to address them. In other consortia, these needs were not well recognized, or they were recognized late in the initiative after relationships had become strained.

- Evidence abounds that community participation in CBPH activities at the coalition or site level was high, and that many residents engaged in various educational skill building and community development forums. Mini-grants to community citizen groups, direct funding of neighborhood organizations for specific work, and community health worker training programs were three of the more successful capacity-building strategies employed.

- Building the capacity of community members to engage, with their partners, in institutional change efforts – in particular, in public health systems change – was romanticized by some stakeholders. Members of the cluster evaluation team felt that most community partners needed more structured learning opportunities and more technical assistance in both types of capacity building if they were to accomplish systems change goals.

### How did participation in the CBPH Initiative affect the capacity of member organizations to carry out their consortia missions?

- The 67 organizations involved in the CBPH Initiative all started at various points on two developmental paths: (1) one leading inward and involving changes in organizations to better support and sustain a CBPH mission, and (2) the other leading outward and involving the capacity to work collaboratively with other organizations and sectors.

- Of the three sectors, academe was able to most clearly identify internal system change goals. These goals involved such things as redefining research protocols to better involve community members; examining the basis for tenure, promotion, and merit awards; revising curriculum; and enhancing students' field

93

experiences. Capacity-building needs for CBOs were quite varied, but often they involved such things as leadership and board development, building community representation, and acquiring strategic planning and proposal writing expertise. Internal system change goals for public health practice agencies were the least well defined, but some partners made radical "cultural shifts" in their working relationships with CBOs on such things as community assessment, health promotion, and disease prevention programs.

- Some of the most important "cultural shifts" that did occur in academe and public health practice were also the hardest to measure. For example, changes involved not only *recognizing* community assets and knowing how to partner towards an immediate goal, but *employing* that knowledge in every core public health function, or throughout a curriculum, or research agenda, or in setting policy at a local or regional level.

- Success in moving systems was highly influenced by the context and history in which consortia operated. Schools building on previous efforts, or in which faculty enjoyed greater support for community-based teaching and research, were able to proceed farther and faster than schools with little tradition in this area, or schools whose faculty were highly dependent on external funding for salary support. Agencies of public health practice varied also in their contexts and constraints. Most were visibly taxed by continuous budget cuts and reorganization due to the advent of managed care.

- While only two of the seven consortia experienced significant systems change in all three sectors, much was attempted and much was accomplished, given the relatively short time frame of the initiative and the difficulty of changing large, bureaucratic systems by using a "bottom-up" strategy. More progress might have been attained in public health education if that had been more clearly understood as the main goal of the initiative. Attempting comprehensive change in all three sectors simultaneously proved to be a highly ambitious goal.

## How did participation in the CBPH Initiative affect the capacity of consortia members to inform policy discussions?

- The answer to this question depends on how one defines policy. From the cluster evaluation team's perspective, participation in the CBPH Initiative did not appear to improve the capacity of consortia to inform *health* policy discussions at the regional, state, or national levels during the active period of implementation (1992-96). It failed to do so for several very understandable reasons. Informing policy discussions was generally not perceived by participants to be a central, or even timely goal during most of the initiative. Additionally, the ability to identify and work on policy issues presumed a level of collaboration that most consortia had not achieved by the fourth year. The policy concerns that did emerge tended to focus (quite logically) on things that affected individual neighborhoods, such as water rights or incinerator waste, or on timely institutional policies affecting academe. Additionally, the knowledge, skills, and experience needed by most members to inform policy discussions were not "budget items." Therefore, in looking across the initiative, and after much in-depth interviewing, we were unable to see how these skills were being acquired or enhanced in any systematic way.

- The CBPH Initiative's National Policy Task Force, which was created in 1994 at the beginning of the third year, did succeed, however, in generating by 1996 wide support among CBPH participants for a document that embraced CBPH principles. It also outlined a broad arena of activity. The Task Force established a working group to explore the development of a new organizational structure to further promote CBPH principles. In 1997, the working group recommended the creation of a new organization (W.K. Kellogg Foundation, 1997, p. 5).

## For individual members and organizations involved, did the benefits of participation in the CBPH Initiative outweigh the costs?

- Despite the challenges, a majority of individual members (64 percent of survey respondents) felt the benefits of participation outweighed the costs. The personal and professional development that occurred, the social and political relationships that developed, and the opportunity to work on projects that members believed in and cared deeply about were all perceived as benefits. Costs were related to the amount of time the partnership took and the stress of intra-consortium conflict.

- Leaders of member organizations were very similar to individual members in their appraisal of the costs and benefits of this experience. If anything, leaders were even more positive (73 percent said the benefits outweighed the costs). Primary benefits were felt in the social and political areas, and the opportunity to advance a mission that was important to their organizations.

- The CBPH philosophy is extremely durable. We believe this philosophy, and members' various and idiosyncratic ways of putting it into practice, will be sustained in coming years. Interestingly, members' commitment to a "CBPH-way of doing business" may be stronger than their commitment to belonging to a particular consortium. As seen in the cost/benefit surveys of 1994 and 1996, the perceived benefits were much higher in some consortia than others. In fact, costs and benefits varied more by which consortium a member belonged to, than which sector (i.e., community, academe, or public health practice) a member represented.

## Lessons Learned

In the year immediately following the fourth and final year of CBPH implementation, I was invited to reflect on the broader lessons learned about community-based programming in health and about cluster evaluation in general with two other evaluators who had been employed by the Foundation for similar initiatives. We found, perhaps not surprisingly, some common lessons learned in three areas (Schmitz, Henry, and Perlstadt, 1997). These areas concerned the importance of: (1) identifying the underlying assumptions for an initiative, and using "program logic," or "theory-based evaluation" (Weiss, 1995) to guide programming; (2) defining more explicitly the definitions and roles for "community" and "community-based programming;" and (3) supporting strong governance and shared leadership. The following reflections about the CBPH Initiative clearly relate to those three overarching areas.

## Holistic Problem Definition and Multiple Goals

One of the conundrums of the CBPH effort was that its greatest asset was also its Achilles' heel. Throughout CBPH there was discussion about the need to overcome categorical funding of public health research, education, and practice. This call was based on a growing consensus that many health and social problems, artificially segregated for the purpose of management or budgeting, are interconnected and experienced in their totality by people in communities. Thus, for example, the physical environment and personal health are interrelated; poverty and illness are inextricably linked. The professional mission in the public health sector is to assure the conditions by which people can be healthy. Those conditions unfortunately do not fall into neat categories in the classic sense. Breaking down the barriers between the disciplines and putting diverse professions together with community folk were deliberate strategies. They were conscious manifestations of the CBPH Initiative's paradigm to define public health problems holistically.

The dilemma is this: Seeing problems holistically, rather than categorically, can be philosophically enlightening, but managerially maddening. Isolated as a limited set of variables, the problems are easier to attack, but depth and scope are sacrificed in the process. Yet holistic problem definition creates an overwhelming agenda for problem solvers in local organizations and the community. Problems such as the disparity in health between higher- and lower-income people must still be broken down into manageable pieces. Some linear planning has to be done. The "doable task" has to be identified and given priority over others, and a rationale for sequencing steps created. The underlying theoretical model of the CBPH Initiative was a good beginning, but the model was quite general. It was not meant to serve, and it could not serve, as a blueprint for reengineering community life and relationships between partnering sectors. Most consortia struggled to redraw the model to make it more workable. Difficult lessons were learned when it came time to translate the very powerful rhetoric of the CBPH philosophy into concrete work plans. As a result, multiple and sometimes conflicting goals continued to coexist, despite lack of time, money, or people to work on them.

95

# Who Comes to the Partnership Table?

The CBPH experience suggests that much of the success of collaboration can be predicted based on the individuals and organizations that initially come to a partnership table. Deciding whom to bring to the partnership table is therefore a critical step. While much has been said about the difficulty of defining community, and the ability of any single person or group to accurately represent "the" community, the problem applies to other sectors as well. Who should represent the university, or the public health department? While these latter institutions may be easier to define, in contrast to the community, finding the right unit (school? department?) and spokesperson to represent even these institutions is not easy.

In a "systems change" initiative, the selection of member organizations and community constituencies and their representatives is especially critical. By contrast, if a university is simply looking for community sites in which to train students, the definition of community is less important; most definitions will suffice. This is because students can learn from a wide variety of contexts, and every community has needs and resources to be tapped. When the primary goal is service learning and augmenting community services, then representative participation is not necessarily a central issue. (It should be noted that the CBPH approach rejected this simpler "outreach" approach to training.)

Because CBPH was conceived as a systems change initiative, the selection of organizations, the definition of community, and the identification of "valid representatives" all became important issues. Some of the decisions were politically charged – and contested. For example, some groups were willing to accept school personnel or social action agency staff as members of "the community." Others were not, unless these individuals were also members of the primary beneficiary group (e.g., persons of color, residents of a poor neighborhood). The definition of community became controversial because in a systems change initiative, more money tends to be on the table, expectations are higher, and the potential consequences greater.

In what ways are consequences greater? Let us consider some examples. If the way an organization "does business" means changing employment eligibility or job status, job functions, or resource allocations, or if new goals challenge core beliefs about the nature of the world, then the approach to selection, definition, and identification becomes critical from a strategic and

political point of view. If not done with diplomacy and clear-sightedness, the process can yield adverse outcomes. Naively inviting the most easily contacted community representatives to the table, for example, can destabilize relationships between community groups. Assigning a junior faculty member the role of representing a department or whole university and expecting him or her to lead the way in tenure reform can place that member in an untenable position.

Significant time and attention needs to be given, therefore (both by funders and proposal writers), to the process of forming partnerships aimed to change systems. The process itself may require outside facilitation if the initiative is new and the sectors do not have a positive history of working together. The process also deserves analysis within the context of the larger ecosystem being addressed. For example, to change the health of underserved populations and invite their representatives to collaborate with academic institutions and public health practice agencies – but not the medical delivery or insurance systems – is to set up something less than a "community of solution." The selection of organizations, the definition of community, and the identification of representatives should be done strategically and carefully and based on a deep understanding of the system or policy being addressed.

# Pairing a Capacity-Building Approach with Systems Change Goals

As stated earlier, member organizations began the initiative with varying levels of capacity for carrying out a CBPH mission. The capacity-building needs of many participating organizations, CBOs, and individuals were underestimated. The challenge of pairing a capacity-building approach with a system change initiative therefore became quite apparent. The challenge was felt by many, and often expressed as "four years is too short a time" to address the goals of changing systems and policy. Even if the goals had been scaled down to local systems change, limited to one sector and a smaller subset of goals, many of the community and institutional partners might still have needed more focused effort before they could have functioned effectively to inform policy discussions.

This finding underscores the need for an appropriate fit between participants and the goals of the initiative. This fit has to be clear from the beginning for the initiative to succeed. Capacity building (especially at the community level) seemed to be the sanctioned goal during the first two years. When more systems change goals were encouraged as priorities in the third year, many consortium members became concerned. They weren't ready to be judged on the extent to which changes might occur at the national, regional, state, or even local levels. With some notable exceptions, the CBPH Initiative did not anticipate the different capabilities needed to inform policy discussions or foster institutional change.

# The Challenge of Shared Leadership and Collaborative Governance

The importance of leadership and strategic process skills for productive partnerships cannot be overstated. Despite the investment of time and resources in the preliminary Leadership and Model Development (LMD) year (as described in Chapter I of this book), many consortia had uneven and often limited levels of leadership knowledge and skills. Some of the leaders were also quite new to public health concepts and issues. Most participants did not have the opportunity to attend LMD sessions. Of the 500 people who became engaged in the initiative during the 1992-96 period, only about 60 (12 percent) participated in one or more LMD sessions during the planning year (1991-92). Given the growth and turnover in membership, there were second and third generations of CBPH participants. Thus, the cluster evaluation team often heard members express the need for "continuing LMD"-type opportunities. On the other hand, some consortia were blessed with exceptional leadership and acquired a wisdom about shared governance that was quite impressive.

It is important to note that even the most gifted leadership from faculty, staff, and community leaders is insufficient for systems change and informing policy discussions unless policymakers and mid- and upper-level administrative agencies also are involved. The idea that change comes only from the "bottom up" (a precept that many listeners took from John McKnight's teaching) needs to be corrected, as it inaccurately reflects seasoned CBPH wisdom and experience. Some very effective change comes from the top and from outside the institutions or sectors. Successful CBPH leaders we interviewed credited supportive deans and directors, and sometimes favorable political figures or contextual events, as supplying the catalytic support to move forward.

# Recommendations for Community-Based Initiatives

On the theory that many readers like to know what travelers would do differently on the next journey, or what they would recommend to others walking a similar road, this chapter concludes with eight recommendations offered by the three directors of cluster evaluations mentioned previously (Schmitz, Henry, and Perlstadt, pp. 32-33). These comments have implications for funders and cluster evaluators, project directors, and project evaluators.

1. **Continue to use planning or visioning phases prior to launching major initiatives.** These are enormously fruitful experiences for people. During this period much critical groundwork is laid in terms of relationships, philosophical grounding, education and training, and positioning resources for action.

2. **Use multiple strategies to support partnership organizations during implementation.** Recognize that consortia represent "moving targets." Because their membership and foci are likely to change over time, they need continuous interaction and support to stay relatively in tune and on the same page of music.

3. **Take the time to build clear theories of action with informed audiences and key stakeholder groups before launching a large-scale policy or systems change initiative.** Involve cluster evaluators and other professional support staff at this stage to research the empirical basis of evidence for the program's "logic model." Use the analysis of the system as a guide for defining the "community" and the sectors that need to be represented. Use the logic models as tools for communication and accountability, and teach partnerships how to do the same.

4. **Clarify whether initiatives are essentially capacity building in nature vs. systems change initiatives.** Consider the implications of the focus for grantee selection, coalition formation, realistic goals and expectations, timelines, and support strategies. If systems change oriented, define the targets or agenda early and often. If capacity building is the intent, connect the capacities to be developed with clear short-term and intermediate milestones, not just a broad, long-term goal.

5. **Clarify what is meant by "community" and "community-based" for a given initiative.** If appropriate, be clear with grantees as to which def-

initions can be considered faithful to the intention of the initiative, and which are not. Enforce agreed-upon rules for community representation.

6. **Consider when and how collaborative partnerships can be instrumental for success, and when this strategy is optional.** Don't expect vulnerable neighborhoods and overworked bureacracies to form new partnerships every time a new initiative is launched. Among other alternatives, consider building the capacity of existing partnerships so they can address problems of their own choice; selecting mature coalitions to play strategic roles in a policy change initiative; allowing grantees to propose a partnership strategy as they see fit.

7. **Don't underestimate the challenge of changing health status, "systems," or of building capacity in communities and institutions.** These are all major endeavors that require long-term funding and short-term milestones to help grantees mark their accomplishments and reflect on their progress.

8. **Build leadership capacity across multiple sectors.** Teach shared leadership skills, which include collaboration, conflict resolution skills, and multicultural competency, among other things. Don't assume that people of color have multicultural skills simply because they are of color, or that people working in institutions don't have them simply because they may not live in distressed neighborhoods.

Engineering capacity-building and systems change initiatives using a community-based approach remains a valid, important endeavor – one that is probably not well-suited for the faint-hearted, however, given its challenges. The eight guidelines above are not formulas or prescriptions that guarantee success. They represent best advice hewn from very honest attempts to see the "whole picture" of these wonderful, complicated, and very powerful initiatives.

# Acknowledgments

The author wishes to acknowledge the entire CBPH cluster evaluation team that produced the work summarized here, especially Carol McGee Johnson, Arthur Himmelman, and Marijo Wunderlich. Much of the present text draws from our annual and final reports, coauthored by the team. I also wish to thank Melanie Petereson Hickey, who served as site visit consultant for one of the consortia. Credit also goes to the CBPH graduate student support staff: Cecilia Goetz, Dung Truong, and Carolyn Link Carlson.

# References

Millett R. *W.K. Kellogg Foundation Cluster Evaluation Model of Evolving Practices.* Battle Creek, MI: W.K. Kellogg Foundation Evaluation Unit; 1995.

Patton MQ. *Utilization-Focused Evaluation* (3rd ed.). Newbury Park, CA: Sage Publications; 1997.

Sanders J. Cluster evaluation. In E Chelimsky and W Shaddish (eds.) *Evaluation for the 21st Century.* Newbury Park, CA: Sage Publications; 1997.

Schmitz CC, Henry R, Perlstadt J. *View From the Balcony: Observations on Programming From Three Cluster Evaluations for the W.K. Kellogg Foundation Health Goal Group.* Minneapolis, MN: University of Minnesota, Center for Urban and Regional Affairs; 1997.

Schmitz CC, Johnson CM, Himmelman A, Wunderlich M. *Cluster Evaluation of the Community-Based Public Health Initiative: 1996 Annual Report and Final Summary.* Minneapolis, MN: University of Minnesota, Center for Urban and Regional Affairs; 1996.

Weiss C. Nothing as practical as good theory: Exploring theory-based evaluation for comprehensive community initiatives for families and children. In JP Connel, AC Kubisch, LB Schorr, and CH Weiss (eds.) *New Approaches to Evaluating Community Initiatives.* New York: Aspen Institute; 1995.

W.K. Kellogg Foundation. *CBPH News* (May 15th). Battle Creek, MI; 1997.

# Chapter X

# Taking a Community-Based Public Health Approach: How Does it Make a Difference?

*Thomas Allen Bruce, Steven Uranga McKane,*
*and Roslyn McCallister Brock*

## Introduction

It is difficult to report on the Community-Based Public Health (CBPH) Initiative in a neutral fashion given our roles as W.K. Kellogg Foundation program officers during the initiative, and since, in many ways, we were changed personally by what we learned and experienced. However, CBPH lessons, observations, and conclusions will nonetheless be reported in this chapter as objectively as possible to share information about how philanthropy can facilitate development in the field of community health.

There are two clusters of data available to inform the field: (1) information about individual CBPH project outcomes and (2) information concerning the overall initiative. This chapter will offer relatively little on the former – in many ways the richest information on CBPH outcomes. (Individual project accomplishments merit a separate report – in particular, the stories captured in print and on videotape of the life-changing events that grew out of the local projects. The Center for the Advancement of Community Based Public Health, created to carry on the work of the CBPH Initiative, plans to publish these stories under the title *Crown of Jewels: Success Stories in Community-Based Public Health*.) Rather, our focus will be on the initiative overall and the lessons it holds for philanthropy, public health, academe, and communities. We will examine the impact of the CBPH Initiative, and detail how it has made a difference to the field and to the diverse partners involved in the process.

## How Did the CBPH Initiative Make a Difference? Definitions

The CBPH Initiative caused us to reexamine some basic definitions and assumptions about health itself and the public health field. To a degree, the readiness by which the individual consortia adopted these new definitions might be considered the first evidence as to *how* a community-based approach has made a difference.

### *What is public health?*

Admittedly, it can be a confusing term. There is the public health system within the health sector, with its focus on whole communities and societies. Because of that, some people call public health the "population" specialty. Then there is the public health emphasis on protecting society from health risks such as environmental pollution and epidemics that are beyond personal control, and promoting better health habits (advocating that we adopt more health-conscious approaches to living). Some people thus call public health the "prevention" specialty.

There is public health as a discipline and many subdisciplines within the field. Some are professions in the classic sense, where graduate education and training are required, leading to specialty certification – preventive medicine, public health nursing, public health dentistry, sanitarians, environmentalists, public health educators, epidemiologists, maternal-child health specialists, public health nutritionists, public health administrators, and public health laboratory technicians. Most public health workers are not educated at the graduate professional level, however, and their careers are formed through an apprentice-like approach to training. Examples are the animal and vector control workers, restaurant and food service inspectors, assistants in management and health finance, lay health planners and health policy analysts, most public health communications personnel, and community health outreach workers.

There is the issue of sponsorship. Public health agencies are publicly supported or function as governmental units, rather than as a part of the personal care health system which is a mix of a few publicly-supported organizations and a great number of private doctors, private clinics and hospitals, managed care plans, and the like. In today's health care marketplace this is changing somewhat, and public health agencies are beginning to enter the field of commerce in some innovative ways as they try to find mechanisms to carry out their public health responsibilities in the face of governmental cutbacks.

Finally, there is the issue of ends or desired outcomes – improved health for all the people ("the public's health" perhaps says it better than "public health"), as opposed to better health care services for individuals and families. Dr. C. Everett Koop said it succinctly: "Health care is vital to all of us some of the time, but public health is vital to all of us all of the time" (1994).

The Institute of Medicine defined public health as: "*The fulfillment of society's interest in assuring the conditions in which people can be healthy*" (1988, p. 7). The CBPH Initiative's goal was to achieve this definition by linking public health educators and practitioners to people in communities who face public health issues every day of their lives.

### How does one define health?
Health clearly is more than just the absence of disease. We sometimes like to think of a healthy person as someone who has a great cushion or reserve built up to avoid becoming ill or unhealthy. The literature speaks often of people in the bloom of health or bursting with good health.

Being vulnerable to illness is likely to be just as important a condition as the state of illness – more so, many in the prevention field would say. As one considers those conditions that allow people to be healthy, it becomes apparent that health must not be limited to a medical connotation. People in direst poverty who struggle every day for survival have very high rates of illness, and it would be hard to say that even those who are not ill are actually healthy. Teenagers who experiment with drugs, guns, sex, and lawlessness cannot be considered healthy when they are so much at risk. Older people, vulnerable anyway, who are forced to live in housing that is unsafe and unsanitary cannot be considered to be healthy under those conditions. A true state of health can thus be equated with a low or reasonably low risk of ill health, and the term "well-being" is commonly used in that context.

For practical purposes, the following definition of health has been used in the CBPH Initiative: *A personal or community condition that reflects the fullest attainment and expression of physical, mental, environmental, spiritual, and economic potential.*

### How does one define community?
There are many definitions of community, and entire books have been written about the various concepts. Few of the books agree. The most common use is a geographic one, so that people who live in a neighborhood or an entire city/town/region are the target of some program or activity. Another frequent use is a group identity around a common theme or issue, such as a community of elders, a gay community, or the Republican Party community.

Although CBPH participants adopted their own definitions of community, the Kellogg Foundation guided their thinking by saying priority in the selection process would be given to consortia that included communities with an especially challenging array of public health problems. A geographic definition was invariably chosen, but the geographic boundaries varied in size from one public housing unit in Atlanta to selected sites/groups/areas throughout Western Massachusetts. Most community sites were characterized by poverty, lack of educational achievement, and high unemployment; many were minority communities with people of color as the consortium representatives.

It became common during the initiative to think of the project's universe as having two major groups, those who were community people, and those who were *not* community people, but functioning within institutions. Such a polarization had some practical realities, but it also had the potential for becoming divisive.

Early on the CBPH Initiative adopted the old adage of community development: *Start where the community is, and move at its pace.* The desire was to find and link with people where they work, play, and gather, rather than trying to create new organizations. The most common gathering sites are churches, schools, clubs, playgrounds, and the community-based organizations found in every neighborhood. One of the difficult lessons for us was discovering that many of these organizations did not understand the CBPH philosophy. They were "service," not "representative," organizations and often as limited as other institutions in understanding the potential of vulnerable people to define and solve their own problems. It was a discovery for many of these groups that community people could bring strong assets to a collaborative endeavor, including a relevant history, knowledge, and the ability to relate positively to decision makers. We also learned that some community organizations ready to partner with prominent institutions run the risk of losing their credibility in the community and connections with constituents.

An awkward problem never fully resolved was the extent to which targeted communities should open their boundaries to include groups that did not have poverty or being "underserved" as a defining issue. With the goal of building the capacity of communities to address public health issues, it clearly was not in their best interest (or their CBPH partners' interest) to bring in individuals and groups accustomed to wielding money, power, and influence to achieve their own objectives. Throughout the initiative an ongoing debate considered whether leadership should try to "empower" affiliated communities through a capacity-building process, or whether they already were sufficiently empowered – needing only more information to justify becoming fully engaged in CBPH programs.

Over many months we discussed various solutions to defining who was in, and who was out, of a given community. Kellogg Foundation staff and many others wanted to be expansive in the definition, and explored using the concept of a community of solution, e.g., all who brought something to help address local community problems or issues were welcome to call themselves members of that community if they wished. Late in the project it became an expressed goal of the national initiative that affiliated institutional partners would become identified as *bona fide* parts of the targeted community, thus effectively adopting the community of solution model. However only in rare instances was this ideal goal ever realized.

The Center for the Advancement of Community Based Public Health has created its own definition of community: *A group of people, regardless of location, geographic proximity, or socioeconomic characteristics, who are linked together by common values, interests, traditions, culture, or geography.*

### How does one define community-based?

The phrase "community-based" is used very commonly today, particularly in the human services sector. It most commonly means community-*placed* or community-*located* programs or services. Another related phrase is community-*oriented*, implying a professionally-driven program that is aimed at, or focused on, some community group. The CBPH Initiative, with its strong emphasis on the validity of community voices in reaching new and better solutions, wanted a more focused, stronger definition. We therefore used the phrase community-*based* as synonymous with community-*rooted*, community-*driven*, community-*spawned*, or community-*owned*. It is entirely in sympathy with a grassroots or bottoms-up approach, although the definitions did not preclude carrying out programs that had both top-down (professional/organizational) and bottom-up approaches. Community-*placed* means, effectively, that one is providing services or carrying our programs *for* and *to* the community, whereas community-*based* means the same activities are *with*

and *by* the community. The definition is a major shift from a *client* mindset to one of partnership and coequal responsibility for activities carried out.

## How Did the CBPH Initiative Make a Difference? General Issues

In the course of the first planning year, the CBPH Initiative began to take on a life of its own. As originally conceived, the primary purpose was to improve the education and training of public health students and other health professionals. Placing that training in the real world of public health practice quickly shifted the center of attention to communities and consortium partners since the quality of that experience would determine what students learned. Much of the energy of the initiative was therefore diverted into community-building activities, since the people in the targeted communities were not initially prepared to serve as tutors and mentors for public health trainees.

Once CBPH communities got a taste of their potential as equal partners in the CBPH Initiative, they began to see the value of leveraging community assets to address other longstanding problems. There was a groundswell of enthusiasm for tackling some of these challenges, and community leaders began moving in a number of directions to capitalize on their newfound insights. The number of partners in the initiative increased considerably as a result of this enthusiasm. Table I shows the expanded number of partners in each of the consortium sites during Year 3, compared with the number of initial partners.

Growth was not universally considered to be positive. At times the CBPH Initiative seemed to provide legitimacy for some aggressive attempts at community activism, and this dampened the support of some of the more conservative partners. On occasion the leadership was even accused by some purists of deserting the original goals of educational enhancement within the public health field.

Perhaps a more valid criticism was that as it evolved CBPH tried to become all things to all people – and in trying for so much it diluted its potential for addressing primary goals. But we would argue that educational outcomes were enhanced, not diluted, by attention to community partners in particular, and to a lesser degree, practice partners. Admittedly, the duration was too short and the financial resources too small for the broad range of community development activities that were initiated through CBPH. This led to some disillusionment on the part of consortium partners as the funding period drew to a close.

# Table I
# Community–Based Public Health Consortia

| State | Public Health Agency | Public Health School | Other Health Schools | Community-Based Organizations |
|---|---|---|---|---|
| **California** | Alameda County Health Care Services Agency | UC Berkeley School of Public Health | UC San Francisco School of Medicine | 21 neighborhood groups; 7 youth groups; 16 CBOs in East 14th Crossroads area of City of Oakland |
| **Georgia** | Fulton Co. Health Dept. Cobb Co. Board of Health | Emory Univ. Rollins School of Public Health | Morehouse School of Medicine | Rose Garden Hills; Kennesaw Village; Fort Hill; and Roosevelt Circle – all in Marietta, GA; initially two public housing units in Atlanta |
| **Maryland** | Baltimore City Health Dept. | School of Hygiene and Public Health, Johns Hopkins Univ. | Johns Hopkins Univ. Schools of Nursing and Medicine | Clergy United for Renewal of East Baltimore (CURE); Heart, Body & Soul; Health Care for the Homeless; Baltimore City Public Schools; The Family Place; The Julie Center |
| **Massachusetts** | Mass. Assoc. of Boards of Health; Mass. Dept. of Public Health | UMass School of Public Health and Health Sciences | UMass Medical School Dept of Family Medicine | Holyoke Latino Community Coalition; Northern Berkshire Community Coalition; Worcester Latino Coalition; North Quabbin Community Coalition |
| **Michigan** | Detroit Health Dept. Genesee Co. Health Dept. | Univ. of Michigan School of Public Health | Univ. of Michigan School of Social Work; Wayne State Univ. School of Social Work; Univ. Detroit-Mercy School of Health Sciences; Univ. of Mich.-Flint | Agape House of Hartford Memorial Baptist Church; Barton McFarlane Neighborhood Assoc.; National Center for Advancement of Blacks in the Health Professions; Flint Odyssey House; Genesee Area Skill Center; Genesee County CAA; Flint Area Community Economic Development; Flint Neighborhood Coalition |
| **North Carolina** | Chatham Co. Health Dept. Orange Co. Health Dept. Wake Co. Health Dept. Lee Co. Health Dept. | Univ. of N.C. at Chapel Hill School of Public Health | UNC at Chapel Hill Area Health Education Centers | Joint Orange-Chatham Community Action; Orange-Chatham Comprehensive Health Services; Wake Health Services; Strengthening the Black Family, Inc. |
| **Washington** | Seattle-King County Health Dept.; Whatcom Co. Health Dept. | Univ. of Wash. School of Public Health & Community Medicine | Univ. of Wash. School of Nursing | Seattle Urban Health Alliance; Lummi Cedar Project; Group Health Cooperative of Puget Sound |

## How Did the CBPH Initiative Make a Difference? Academic Issues

The challenge for the academic partners was to take advantage of community and practice partnerships to change the way business was usually done. Since the university's primary missions are education, research, and service, each of these areas needed to be reexamined within the context of lessons learned from the CBPH Initiative. The problem for many of the health professions schools was that they had too few faculty members with knowledge or experience in community health issues. Most faculties had many years ago abandoned or reduced their community education programs because of the belief that apprentice-style learning was inferior to modern classroom and laboratory teaching. Most faculty members had been schooled in professional specialty areas removed from either practice or community service venues.

To their credit, most of the schools of public health that were members of the national consortia responded well to the challenge. Affiliated schools of nursing were generally outstanding in their performance, and schools of medicine played an active role. Some of the academic achievements were:

- 31 new CBPH-related courses were put in place in the involved schools.

- 51 courses were revised to increase the community content.

- 3,000 students were involved in classroom instruction on community-based approaches.

- 1,500 students were placed in internships or field sites to explore community-based concepts.

- 22 new faculty (including many people of color) were recruited from the targeted communities.

- 66 new staff were recruited from the targeted communities.

- 3 schools of public health established a new faculty position to direct community-based instruction.

- 750 faculty and staff received supplementary training in community-focused teaching and/or research.

- 3 schools of public health created new promotion/tenure criteria to facilitate academic work in communities.

- 3 schools implemented community-based research protocols.

- 50 or more CBPH-related academic papers were published.

- $20 million in new grant funds were leveraged to sustain CBPH-related activities.

By the final year, four major principles appeared to be of fundamental importance in the pursuit of community-based teaching and research:

1. A broad definition of *health* is needed, and indeed lies at the heart of the CBPH philosophy.

2. High values for *diversity* are warranted, and understanding multicultural approaches is an essential element of carrying out public health programs.

3. An understanding of the *processes of community organization and development* are fundamental to implementing the CBPH philosophy.

4. An *asset approach* rather than a deficit or needs approach needs to be incorporated into the core curriculum of public health programs.

We learned that multiple voices increase the likelihood that public health policy will be relevant, as it is taught and practiced within academic centers. We saw also that the pace of change and adaptation within academic centers themselves could be accelerated by community input and by the challenges of responding to community concerns.

Cluster evaluation added to a general understanding of the many elements involved in each academic institution's development toward CBPH principles. Some steps are easy to accomplish; others are infinitely more difficult. Table II shows the ladder of increasing complexity for academic centers in the last column.

The list of curricular competencies in community-based public health, as developed by the Johns Hopkins University School of Public Health in conjunction with some other CBPH partners, can be found in Appendix A.

## How Did the CBPH Initiative Make a Difference? Practice Issues

The challenge for public health agencies was to become more mission-driven and to improve the health outcomes of their populations. The goal was far more ambitious than simply generating additional community services, however valuable they might be to the targeted communities. Given the challenge, some CBPH agency partners never got beyond that first step.

103

The practice challenges of the initiative were to work in genuine partnership with the academic and community partners in order to carry out the three core public health functions of assessment, policy development, and assurance. But to fulfill the CBPH vision, these had to be carried out in vastly different ways than had been done in the past. *Assessing* the health issues and needs of the community had to be done in tandem with partners, and within the context of defining community assets available to deal with the problems identified. *Developing policies* to present strategic alternatives to decision makers about best ways to address health problems also had to be done in conjunction with community partners and the academic specialists, and the policies needed to grow out of the real-world experiences of attempted community health interventions. Finally, trying to *assure* that the public's health needs could be met required the constant input of informed and engaged consortium partners who had their own ideas of how to guarantee results.

At the conclusion of the CBPH Initiative, some of the practice achievements were:

1. Public health practice was defined more broadly in all sites, adding a stronger social/cultural context for public health problems.

2. Community partners in all consortia had more voice in decisions about their own local services, and more community persons were recruited and trained to carry out public health functions.

3. Targeted communities received significantly increased access to health services.

In some instances it was possible to see real transformation of the public health agency as a result of its CBPH experiences, and this perhaps is the most illuminating aspect of the initiative's impact. Changes ranged from a complete reorganization of the agency to incorporate community-based principles, to an expanded outreach program, engaging community-based organizations and academic partners in efforts to tackle new community health challenges, to increasing the role of the agency as an advocacy organization for broadly integrated community development.

Some specific manifestations of CBPH impact on individual agencies and their partners include:

• One agency added a new community to the project from its own budget, and brought in other consortium partners to facilitate the training that was needed by local people.

• Two agencies trained community health workers and supervised their work; in one community the focus was on screening for tuberculosis, diabetes, and eye problems.

• One agency launched a Male Responsibility Clinic within an urban public housing complex.

• One agency shifted its entire mission to a community focus.

• One agency expanded its number of community links to address local health priorities.

• One agency expanded its territory of responsibility to include a nearby tribal reservation.

• One agency organized 23 community focus groups to redefine its programs, then restructured itself to reflect its new direction.

Despite these encouraging strides in public health practice, some dilemmas remained at the end of the funding period. Local agencies were the most difficult of the three partners to engage in genuine community-based approaches because they were so distracted with other matters. It was common to see personnel and budget shortages, a lack of experience in collaboration, inadequate support from political and/or institutional governance systems, and a general feeling of inadequacy from having insufficient resources to keep up with the flood of requests for assistance to address public health problems. Further, except at the most senior levels, the readiness of public health agency personnel was limited for the types of community engagements that the project demanded. Most staff members were trained only at the task level for focused interventions.

Through CBPH, we reached one dominant conclusion about the role of the local public health agency: it is a critical pathway for connecting people in communities to public health issues and public health professionals. Our major regret was that the CBPH Initiative never truly overcame the service mentality of agency personnel in several sites. Many interpreted being a good CBPH partner as increasing the delivery of established program services (e.g., immunizations, maternal-child care, environmental screening) to targeted communities.

The progressively more difficult steps to incorporating the CBPH vision into practice activities can be seen in the first column of Table II.

## Table II
## Imagining Systems Change in CBPH Institutions and Communities

| Public Health Practice Agencies | Communities | Academic Institutions |
|---|---|---|
| • Development of a new public health mission | • Full power-sharing partnerships with external institutions | • Mission change reflects epistemological change in the definition of public health knowledge, how that knowledge is gained and imparted |
| • Strong advocacy for big picture policy issues surrounding health (e.g., employment, education, environment, universal health coverage) | • Ability to set priorities and control resources around public health, quality of life issues | • Establishment of endowed chairs for researchers, educators, and practitioners of community-based approach to public health |
| • Leadership in bringing policymakers together to address health policy issues | • Positive, proactive ways of addressing institutional and environmental racism | • Tenured appointments for faculty researching, teaching, and practicing a community-based approach |
| • Reorganization of departments, interagency collaborations | • Mutually respective participation with academic and practice partners in research, education, service, outreach, assessment and planning, and other functions | • Publications about community-based public health |
| • Interpreting "public health" broadly, as problems embedded in a context | • Development of community infrastructure; achieving the level of organizational capacity needed to be in power-sharing relationships with institutions | • Recruitment and retention of faculty and students of color |
| • Emphasis on community capacity throughout core functions | • Building career and education pathways for young people | • Research funding for community-based public health |
| • Involvement of community and academic partners in strategic planning for the health department | • Expanded community base, mobilizing volunteers | • Involvement of faculty in public health practice program planning and service |
| • Recruitment and retention of people of color and others from target communities | • Leadership development | • Curriculum planning with practice and community input |
| • Development of village (neighborhood) health workers and outreach staff | • Board development | • Graduate level course revision; development of a core curriculum in community-based public health |
| • Department-wide training on multicultural competencies | • Training and individual skill development in communication, diversity, organization, planning, financial management, citizen politics | • Senior faculty support and mentorship for community-based research, teaching, and service |
| • Contracting services out to neighborhood health agencies | • Working with student interns in the community environment | • Coordination of internship experiences |
| • Working proactively with university interns | | • Revision of existing courses, development of new courses in public health |
| • Linking needs assessments to community assets and capacity building | | • Use of community and practice instructors |
| • Developing a citizen board | | • Expansion of student practica and field experiences |
| • Sharing information, creating feedback loops with community and others | | |

**Level of Systems Change** — High ← → Low

105

## How Did the CBPH Initiative Make a Difference? Community Issues

The challenge for each community was to increase the capacity of its citizens to identify health issues and articulate needs within the context of its own culture and values. Each community group also needed to interact with its two consortium partners in ways that could be mutually helpful. The community representatives at first were unsure about their role in improving community health. Over time, they became informed and engaged in public health action – a dramatic difference from their stance at the outset.

From the perspective of their consortium partners, involving community members in public health teaching, research, and practice was seen as appropriate and beneficial. Community participation allowed the consortia to say and do things that professional organizations could not, and collaboration brought access to a broader range of resources to address public health problems than the communities might have had without their contacts in the partnership.

It was not, however, an easy road for community participants. Those who started with little experience in collaborative projects, and those with low levels of trust in professional partners, tended to move more slowly into genuine partnerships than those with track records of community action. For even the most experienced community groups, moreover, building the capacity for meaningful collaboration could be a long and difficult process. Those individuals who represented poor and vulnerable communities had financial and time barriers to collaboration that limited their ability to contribute – more, for instance, than their professional partners who enjoyed such things as salaried support for planning, time off for meetings, and assigned work responsibilities for public health interventions.

Certainly, the people who live in settings with many public health problems brought unique insight into the causal conditions and interventions needed to improve community health. Perhaps more importantly, they brought ideas about how interventions should be carried out. With the diverse contributions of people in communities and people in institutions – skills, perspectives, and approaches to partnering – solid coalitions were built. More than that, they achieved breakthroughs in addressing notoriously resistant public health problems. And although it may take years to prove that the prevalence of chronic health conditions has been reduced as a result of CBPH consortia efforts, early indicators are in place to measure outcomes.

Some of the ways communities responded to the CBPH Initiative include:

- More than 600 community health workers were recruited, trained, and employed in each of the seven projects – with 230 still actively serving as advocates, technical assistants, or paraprofessionals who are increasing access of local people to health services, or in some instances carrying out community research studies.

- More than 120 community projects for children and youth were undertaken, reaching 10,600 children.

- Overall, 324 community projects reached more than 34,000 people in health improvement and local development programs.

- $3 million in grants were leveraged by community groups for spinoff activities (that is, to support activities of the consortia, rather than supporting the consortia themselves).

- In one urban school system's learn-and-earn program, summer health careers enrollment rose from 11 to 68 over three years, and community placements climbed as traditional hospital placements decreased.

- Health career clubs were formed in one community, and more than 100 scholarships were provided under an urban health alliance.

- A playground was created in a rural township to allow opportunities for immigrant Hispanic youth to know and play with local children, averting the class and race fights that had been developing prior to that time.

- The return to a tribal custom of canoe pulling and racing was implemented on a native reservation in the Pacific Northwest, as a way of averting some growing problems with substance abuse among the youth.

- A neighborhood after-school program for children provided such an impetus for learning that the average level of academic performance in that community went from below average to honors-level achievement.

- An annual careers day program for youth in one community was expanded in numbers and scope to the extent that it became a national model for other such programs around the nation.

- A church-based health promotion program was so successful that it began training ministerial students in addition to the nursing, medical, and public health students who participated in its activities.

- A Latino community-based organization organized three health promotion centers in its community around the issue of HIV/AIDS prevention and treatment.

- Another Latino community-based organization developed an aggressive media campaign for health promotion.

- One community challenged the planned use of funds resulting from the sale of a nonprofit hospital, and was able to persuade the new conversion board that funds should be used for community health improvement rather than for the benefit of a limited few.

- Many community groups launched neighborhood fix-up, clean-up programs; others tackled more substantive issues such as improved water and sewage services for isolated rural homes.

- Several communities became strong advocates for strengthening the local public health system.

The increasingly challenging steps for community advancement in the CBPH approaches can be seen in the middle column in Table II.

## How Did the CBPH Initiative Make a Difference? Consortium Issues

One of the most difficult challenges in assessing the impact of CBPH was determining the role played by the full consortium in achieving each of the outcomes. To some extent, we can only speculate on the degree to which all the partners were involved.

The ideal consortium was not just a three-way linkage between academic, practice, and community entities. It was a partnership between a university group that was committed to the CBPH philosophy in its teaching, research, and service. The academic partner connected with a practice agency that made a major investment in community-based principles and approaches in applying public health programs and services to their constituencies. Both joined informed community-based organizations engaged in health improvements – groups committed to a collaborative endeavor with the academic and practice partners.

It seems doubtful that there were three-way discussions and approaches to every issue that arose during the course of the project. Most often there were sub-projects that involved only two of the partners, or in many instances only one. But the power and influence of the entire CBPH consortium in setting stan-

dards and creating a vision that encompassed all partner activities was a pervasive aspect of the initiative throughout its course. It seems premature then to conclude that complex consortia are not the way to approach future community problem solving.

There were a number of *governance issues* among the various consortia. The kind of governing structure that was created did not seem to be as important as the perception among partners that is was fair and accountable. A carefully designed approach in North Carolina demanded a great deal of time from the members and seemed to work well. In Michigan a far less structured consortium – one with no governing board or bylaws – also functioned effectively through the efforts of a series of overlapping teams. Two consortia went through traumatic changes in their governing structures after the partnerships struggled with resource and power issues. But they were able to resolve differences and come together again in a looser, but no less effective, structure. One consortium had a rather fragile structure that seemed more the result of personal bonds and pledges than any true governance arrangement, but it too was effective.

What is remarkable is that in spite of these structural variations and the lack of experience of so many participants, the consortia achieved so much. Stories from the CBPH Initiative abound about how each of the partners was humbled by the experience, how each one had to learn to listen to the others, how each one was strengthened and empowered by the new insights that grew out of adversity and unexpected success.

*Individual leadership* was evident at every level of CBPH work, and in every consortium. The senior cadre of leaders for the overall initiative was identified and trained during the Leadership and Model Development year, and it was a mistake not to have continued this period of training at each of the sites. New leaders emerged over time, and in different contexts. In some instances, professionals from academic institutions were the mainstay of the consortia. Some of the health departments also had strong natural leaders within the project. But in the end it was the community leadership that emerged as exemplary. Many of these leaders blossomed during the period of community enhancement as part of the CBPH partnerships.

*Shared leadership,* as opposed to individual leadership, was also evident throughout the CBPH Initiative. It was not, however, the defining issue of whether the partners were able to collaborate on specific programs, as was suggested in one analysis. The integrated, interconnected nature of each consortium's activities engendered a level of collaboration that created opportunities for sharing information, resources, and skills.

*Learning to access capital, both human and financial,* was an important attribute of CBPH work at each site. Skill building, resourcefulness, entrepreneurial growth, and business savvy increased exponentially through the project – more in some places than others. All projects have approached sustainability in one way or another. Some have turned to other private philanthropic organizations for support; others have started to institutionalize their projects within their own governmental or institutional bureaucracies. Still others have turned to corporate partners, and the California project has been integrated into the local Empowerment Zone alliance. Evidence of the financial progress and the commitment to sustainability has been seen indirectly in the growing sense of comfort across the groups with addressing such challenging and complex issues as social change.

## How Did the CBPH Initiative Make a Difference? Core Lessons

Participants in the CBPH Initiative drew several conclusions from their efforts in working together to improve the public's health. The central lesson was that *community lies at the heart of public health, and the improvement of health is best achieved by full participation of the community in the selection, design, and implementation of programs and services that traditionally have been provided by health professionals.*

Other general CBPH lessons include:

• There is a specific body of knowledge for community-based approaches to public health, and core competencies can be identified.

• A community-based approach is not only possible, but has been shown to advance the goals of public health education and practice.

• Community partnerships with health education institutions can transform and enlighten the usual process of teaching and learning.

• Institutional change is facilitated and enhanced by the involvement of faculty, staff, or administrators with previous experiences in community health development.

## Conclusions

Based on the results, and on our observations and analysis of the CBPH Initiative, we have reached several conclusions related to the utility and promise of community-based approaches. We conclude that taking a community-based approach did make a profound difference in the outcomes of this initiative – differences seen in the changes that occurred in each of the participant groups. We also conclude that the consortium approach to development is a powerful one with great potential for addressing some of society's most complex issues. We believe in the importance of creating a vital role for community voices in decision making related to public health practice and education, however cumbersome the process might seem at the outset. Through the work of CBPH grantees, we have become increasingly convinced that the investments of time, energy, and support needed to connect community, public health practice, and academic pursuits will pay off handsomely in the end. Finally, we believe that community-based approaches, once begun, can be sustained over time without the influx of significant new financial resources.

## References

Koop CE. Speech. Medicine and Public Health Institute. Chicago, IL; July 14, 1994.

Institute of Medicine. *The Future of Public Health.* Washington, DC: National Academy Press; 1988.

# Chapter XI

# A Foundation Perspective on the Community-Based Public Health Initiative

*Gloria R. Smith and Kay Randolph-Back*

When it inaugurated the Community-Based Public Health Initiative in 1991 the W.K. Kellogg Foundation entered unexplored territory with a new theory to test. Today, in light of developments in research and practice in the intervening years, the theory tested in the initiative might be called prescient.

But at the time, what we called internally just "CBPH" was novel enough to be risky and to be difficult to explain to our colleagues and prospective grantees. Foundations can take risks. Social, economic, and public policy in the United States gives foundations the latitude to do this. Indeed, an analogy between foundation grantmaking and for-profit investment in start-up ventures is under discussion today in some circles. One concept is that the investment of venture capital in nonprofit social enterprises should increasingly become a role of philanthropy (Reis and Clohesy, 1999). Sometimes associated with Silicon Valley, the concept's currency is due in part to the emergence of "new" money among young, very entrepreneurial people with fortunes made in technology. Some are motivated to contribute financial resources *and* business acumen to nonprofit ventures for solutions to social problems that aim to get the job done with businesslike efficiency and effectiveness. At the Kellogg Foundation, the long-ingrained concepts of risktaking and of grantmaking as investment come from a different time and context. In striving to determine how to deploy his accumulated wealth wisely, W.K. Kellogg was influenced by a White House Conference on Children and Youth he attended. In 1930 he decided, "I'll invest my money in people."

Foundations have comparatively limited resources with which to make investments. For example, during the first half of the 1990s formal philanthropy (such as private, public, and family foundations) represented only about 12 percent of private giving in the United States and only about 2 percent of funding to the nonprofit sector (sometimes called the third or the independent sector). But for many foundations, including the Kellogg Foundation, those investments are all at the margin of their grantees' work; that is, at the point where a nonprofit entity can try something new, something that is not identical to its ongoing operations. This point – the point of innovation – is the one at which it is *appropriate* to take risks, but the risks should be calculated and based on theory.

This chapter is intended to place the history of CBPH and the current status and future of its core concepts and accomplishments within the context of several apparent drivers of change within our society. We will discuss three aspects of theory and risk in CBPH:

1. The theory in CBPH and two of the discoveries the Foundation made in testing that theory;

2. New research findings that make the theory more than timely today; and

3. Why the real risk in investment in innovation is not the risk of failure, but the risk of success!

## Testing the CBPH Theory – Two Discoveries

### The Theory: The CBPH Partnership Model

In 1986 health programming at the Kellogg Foundation began to evolve toward what eventually became – and remains today – a focus on *partnership between communities and institutions*. The core concept is that *both* communities and institutions, not just institutions alone, have resources and knowledge essential to solving problems. In writing an account of CBPH, we want to emphasize that Foundation staff's thinking, skills, and experience relative to this concept were very much "in development" when CBPH was inaugurated. Indeed, as learners ourselves, we sometimes frustrated our grantees, which they were not shy about reporting to us. Therefore, our reflections back to the time in the development of health programming when CBPH

109

began may well articulate the theory in a way it neither was nor could have been articulated then. Testing the theory entailed not only applying and refining it, but also coming to understand what the theory actually was and what it implied. The authors' intellectual effort, then, is not really to be historical but to synthesize Foundation staff's learning.

The community-institutional partnership appeared in CBPH in a complex variation. A CBPH consortium had three types of partners: institutions of higher education, public health agencies, and local community organizations. Bringing together such disparate types of organizations – the *academic*, *practice*, and *community* partners, as they were called – was a bold move, one that worked, but not without challenges and lessons. The theory posited that each type of partner was *necessary* and no two alone were *sufficient* for reform to occur. The reform sought was in health professions education. Foundation staff shared a view common among experts that, in general, institutions have difficulty transforming from *inside*. The initiative tested the theory that partnering health professions education institutions with *outside, nonacademic* organizations could help the institutions achieve change.

The Foundation's interest in reform was prompted by the decline of public health. This decline was of concern to program staff in their programming direction and professional disciplines. It had been delineated by the Institute of Medicine in its 1988 report, *The Future of Public Health*, which the Foundation had helped to fund. The Foundation chose higher education as the locus of effort for reversing the decline. Higher education appeared to offer both the best entry point and the greatest potential return on investment. The mission in higher education is *education, research, and service*. The effects of incorporating community-based approaches into the mission would reach far, we reasoned, since the educational institutions train new professionals, define the discipline, determine the standard, set the research agenda, and inform the field. The CBPH partnerships were, therefore, to implement new models for *community-based education, research, and service*.

It clearly followed from the theory that local health departments had to be outside partners to the educational institutions. Incorporation of community-based approaches into the mission of academic institutions necessitated their collaborating with health departments in communities.

Threefolding the partnership was felt to be essential even though adding community-based organizations (CBOs) would make the partnering process more difficult. The practice for which the institutions were preparing professionals itself had to be imbued with community-based approaches.[1] The premise was that the discipline of public health had become so disconnected from people and organizations in communities that both health departments and health professions schools needed to partner with CBOs as well as with each other.

For the academicians and the practitioners to learn to partner effectively with communities, the communities had to be strong partners. Weakness would confirm stereotypes that communities were incapable and needy and required the help of academicians and practitioners due to their superior knowledge. If the community partners were not strong, educators and practitioners would not learn how to work in partnerships where communities had real voice.

According to the theory, the models of community-based teaching, research, and service would demonstrate *within and to the professional discipline* that the health of people in communities can be improved when they actively participate in the work of public health. The discipline would develop state-of-the-art skills in facilitating active participation by community members in identifying and solving problems, determining how to allocate scarce resources, establishing priorities, bringing talents to the table, and taking action. And the discipline would reorient academic research toward community participation. Researchers would (1) involve community members in setting the research agenda and conducting the research; and (2) rigorously document and evaluate the outcomes of community-based approaches.

Successful partnership models of community-based teaching, research, and service would have policy significance. Public health had been found to be weak and in decline just when it was needed as a powerful, cost-effective complement to medical care. One promotes the health of populations, while the other treats the illnesses of individuals. *Community-based public health –*

---

[1] A comparison can be made with the Community Partnerships with Health Professions Education Initiative (CP/HPE), which began before CBPH. The CP/HPE Initiative was intended to promote the choice of careers in primary care by medical, undergraduate nursing, and other health professions students. The method used was out-of-hospital, multidisciplinary training in community-based sites. Considerable effort in the initiative went into establishing new sites or further developing existing ones. The initiative demonstrated the basic principle that change had to occur in service delivery simultaneously with change in education. Sites had to be available in communities in order for professionals in training to be educated for community-based practice.

coming into being out of the partnership of professionals in practice, academicians and students in institutions, and people in communities – could strengthen the voice and effectiveness of public health as an important and integral part of the national health system.

The community-institutional partnership was not only the *means* for achieving reform in health professions education, it was the *object* of reform. Partnership was to remain, post-reform, as a new way of doing business in the institutions. That meant, of course, that the institutions would continue to need willing and able partners. Thus, CBPH, while designed as and calling itself a health professions education initiative, implicitly posited that all the partners would change.

### The Discovery of Faculty's Needs for Support

The primary theory that CBPH applied was the partnership theory. We were testing the use of external levers for change by institutions of higher education. The CBPH Initiative's evaluator found that the academic partners made meaningful changes during their participation in the initiative. This finding was part of the evidence that the application of the theory worked; that is, the use, through a partnership structure, of outside organizations as external levers produced positive change in educational institutions.

The partnership theory needed our concentrated attention because the concept (of tripartite community-institutional partnership) was *both* creative *and* difficult to put into practice. But our concentration on organizational levers *outside* an institution meant that we had not given much attention to theory about how change would occur *inside* an institution. One important discovery was the degree of readiness and willingness in some faculty to make changes that would reorient teaching, research, and service toward community-based approaches. Some faculty members were ready for the opportunity CBPH offered. What they did when given the chance was an affirmation of the wisdom of Mr. Kellogg's decision to invest his money in people. These faculty members' readiness and willingness contributed significantly to the formation and management of active, thriving partnerships and to creating a climate for activism in communities. These activities of faculty members also influenced their institutions internally, to differing degrees, and helped to foster the institutional changes in curriculum, incentives for faculty, and other areas documented during the course of the initiative.

We saw that the structure and resources provided by CBPH had supported these faculty and enabled them to move from readiness and willingness to concrete action and results. Their concrete actions had been rewarding, and sometimes also rewarded, in a number of ways. Their skills developed. Their willingness to innovate was reinforced. They made changes. They contributed to change made by others, inside and outside their institutions. And we found it notable that the institutional changes they helped to facilitate included the creation of opportunities for recognition and reward for faculty who incorporated community-based approaches into teaching, research, and service.

Faculty readiness and the results when it was activated by structure and resources had implications for our support of further development of community-based public health. Academic institutions had demonstrated the creation internally of faculty rewards for community-based approaches. A companion action would be our creation of *external* rewards. An external mechanism could be a force for change in other institutions as well as a reinforcement of change in CBPH institutions. An external mechanism for faculty reward could provide another form of structure and support, function as a beacon light for established and new faculty in various venues who might be ready and willing, and enhance the visibility, credibility, and knowledge base for community-based public health within the professional disciplines.

In 1997 the Foundation established its new **Community Health Scholars Program** for the purpose of developing and strengthening emerging faculty's competencies in community-based approaches to teaching, service, and research. The program is increasing the number of faculty members at schools of public health who have community health competencies and are able to meet tenure requirements. The first five scholars were funded in 1998, and a total of 30 will be funded in all. Scholars are prospective or junior faculty who are each awarded a 12-month fellowship and a research fund for postdoctoral study to enhance their understanding of community health determinants, community organizations, and community leadership. Three schools of pub-

> *One important discovery was the degree of readiness and willingness in some faculty to make changes that would reorient teaching, research, and service toward community-based approaches.*

111

lic health were chosen as training sites in the program. All had participated in CBPH. They provide the scholars with access to academic resources, including faculty, and community resources, including partnerships between the universities and community organizations.

## The Discovery of Communities' Capacities and Capabilities

If CBPH *activated* faculty, it *ignited* communities. Hundreds of projects reached tens of thousands of people in the participating communities. The list of all the CBOs involved is long. The initiative evaluator reported that community participation was high, saying "many residents engaged in various educational skill-building and community development forums." The spectrum of activities in the projects was wide and included youth development, career awareness, and community scholarships for children; health education, promotion, and risk-reduction; creation of health promotion and healing centers through the work of community members backed by academic and agency partners; advocacy on health issues in the community; revitalization and civic participation in neighborhoods; incorporation of healthy lifestyle issues in church messages and activities; and recruitment, training, and employment of hundreds of community health workers from the communities.

There were creative efforts to break the mold to achieve genuine community-centeredness. Several communities reached beyond the formal CBO structures to empower residents through mini-grants to grassroots groups. Community-based interventions demonstrated creativity and responsiveness to the context of people's lives. At the Foundation we remarked on the aptness and impact, for example, of one locale's reintroduction of the ancestral tradition of canoe pulling for tribal youth – young people who often face special risks for substance abuse.

The energy, activity, and creativity displayed by the community partners within the CBPH structure were evidence that our theory was on target. The communities were demonstrating their capacities as partners to the academic and agency partners. They were demonstrating the potential for substantial gains in public health to be derived from *forming active working relationships with communities*. The academic and agency partners had the chance to learn that engaged communities

had strength, wisdom, and capacity to contribute to health improvement.

The partnership structure involved communities in order to support their own learning and action, but more importantly in order that they might *teach* their partners. From the Foundation's programming experience with communities in the United States and Latin America, we had the hope, expectation, and confidence that the communities would be energetic, independent, and inventive enough to shake up the natural inertia of the universities and the agencies. *Separate funding* for one consortium's community partner was important to its effectiveness as an independent, outside voice. The surprise for us was that what the communities actually did broke out of the confines erected by our perhaps-limited imaginations and took its own course. The process was not tidy, which added another dimension to managing the complex tripartite partnership structure. It was not only that there were three types of partners, but also that the community partner comprised multiple CBOs, large and small, experienced and inexperienced, sometimes unrelated to each other, sometimes connected to each other, and sometimes in conflict with each other.

*The community partners richly rewarded the academic and agency partners and the Foundation by creating opportunities for real learning.*

The community partners richly rewarded the academic and agency partners and the Foundation by creating opportunities for real learning. In the academic sector our Community Health Scholars Program supports, as noted earlier, further development of learning with and from communities.

In the practice sector the Foundation began an initiative in 1996 to broaden the engagement of communities in the mission of public health. The initiative is **Turning Point: Collaborating for a New Century in Public Health**. The CBPH Initiative evaluators had reported a degree of growth in capacity within the practice sector for providing communities with technical support. Public health agencies had also participated in forming linkages. The evaluators found that "a significant mass of people in all three sectors now have concrete linkages – ideas and strategies – for working together on community-centered projects that build on the assets (not the deficits) of underserved communities." Turning Point affords public health agencies opportunities to grow further in skills, learning, and effectiveness by participating in wider-scope partnerships. Local Turning Point partnerships in 41 communities in 14 states engage organizations from many sectors (public health agencies, businesses, schools, police and fire departments, churches, citizens groups, et cetera) to work together as stakeholders in public health broadly conceived.

While creating opportunities for learning by all, the communities' activism also created tension within the Foundation's initiative management because CBPH was not an initiative for building *community* capacity per se; it was a health professions education initiative that engaged communities as partners in the reform of teaching, research, and service. In some ways the ambiguity was never resolved, a phenomenon that occurs in grantmaking just as it does in other areas of life. But the experience made us better prepared to move forward with Turning Point.

## Timeliness of CBPH Theory Today

New research shows that the health status of the individual is linked not just to personal socioeconomic status — that is, the individual's place in the society and economy — but also to the social and economic structure of the society itself. Probably the most dramatic and compelling finding is that overall population health status in one of the fifty states or in one of the industrialized countries studied varies inversely — when compared with the other states or the other countries, respectively — with the degree of income inequality in the state or country (Kawachi and Kennedy, 1999). All strata of the population are adversely affected by greater income inequality. The groups at the lower end of the income scale are affected more, but all are affected. Income inequality displays a gradient effect in all segments of income distribution in the population.

Taken together with established findings (such as the linkage between poverty and health status), these facts are a reminder that health is not just personally determined by the individual's genes or behavior, or determined by factors in the physical environment that affect entire populations (air and water quality, for instance). It is also determined by society's decisions and choices about the distribution of resources and opportunities.

The beauty of the research on income inequality is the finding that the health of all income groups is affected. This finding buttresses the rationale in Turning Point that everyone has a stake in public health. The implications for improving the health of people — and reducing the reliance on expensive medical treatment as the centerpiece of health services — are extraordinary.

Relationships within the society — person-to-person, group-to-group, sector-to-sector, et cetera — are implicated in the current research findings about income inequality, discrimination and racism, social and workplace status, and other social determinants of health. Interestingly, not all the relevant research is coming from academic researchers. In the United States, corporate sector detailed studies show relative rates of injury, illness, and absence correlated to factors such as whether jobs are high-control or low-control and whether the workplace climate includes such elements as participatory management style.

Although the concept of CBPH grew out of an understanding of the social determinants of health — including the disproportionate control over socially-valued resources vested in academic institutions — the initiative was designed before the first research findings on income inequity were issued. Several aspects of the initiative are relevant to the role of social determinants of health, such as career awareness for youth, youth development to counter hopelessness, and training and employment of community health workers, to mention a few. But the aspect that sets CBPH apart in its relevance to the emerging body of troubling research findings is its concentration on building relationships among a complex of immensely disparate partners. One researcher today states explicitly, "Relationships are primary, all else is derivative" (David, 1998). If relationships are primary to health and well-being and if the primary basis for social determination of health is social and economic relationships, then translating research into remedy will require great skill and good will in bridging social divides and building relationships among disparate groups.

The occasions for people to grasp in a living and practical way (nonsimulated at the electronic hearth and nonsentimental) that we are all in the same policy-boat are not frequent in modern America. Much less do people have the chance to put that insight to work by taking action together. The CBPH Initiative gave its participants that chance, and it created a body of learning on how to cross community-institutional divides. The initiative evaluators were very clear in saying that CBPH had meant much to many participants. This book reflects that fact. The evaluators further observed, "As a capacity-building initiative, ...[CBPH] made tremendous progress in building the capacity of community and academic sectors to partner around the reform of public health research, teaching, and service. ... The initiative made especially strong impact on nurturing community leaders and turning some fledgling CBOs ... into real players in public policy discussions."

## Sustainability, Scale-Up, and Replication – Where the Real Risk of Social Investment Lies

We began this chapter by noting that CBPH was a risky venture. This section elaborates on the nature of risk in grantmaking. The section concludes by mentioning some of the strategies the Kellogg Foundation is trying or considering to meet this risk.

The greatest risk in making a social investment arises not because the undertaking may fail but because it may succeed. Good solutions often do not have wide impact. They die or they remain small, are not institutionalized, are not copied, do not become rooted, are not further developed, and do not inform the field. They do not become nodes for growth and maturation of a community-change process. Success brings new issues and new challenges for both grantmakers and grantees. A project may succeed brilliantly but prove to be grant-dependent and ultimately collapse. Within this framework the grantmaker's risk is not that a project will fail; if it does, those involved can learn, move on, and use the learning from failure for the next venture. The risk arising when a project succeeds is that the infrastructure, skills, adaptability, intention, timeliness, and resources necessary to make the success into something with long-term and widespread impact may not be present.

The philanthropic sector is undergoing change. One source of change is the entry of new resources and new foundations into the field. What is predicted to become an immense transfer of wealth in the United States has begun, and the accumulation of wealth by individuals and families has already resulted in the creation of new foundations and an increase in the corpora of existing foundations. Conversion of nonprofit hospitals, nonprofit Blue Cross/Blue Shield corporations, and other health organizations to for-profit status has also resulted in the creation of new entities called "conversion" foundations.

Whether created through transfer of private wealth or of assets held for public benefit, several of the new foundations are "finding their way" as grantmakers. At the same time, several large, established foundations (including the W.K. Kellogg Foundation) are seeking to

work more strategically to deploy their resources in a way that will produce greater and more lasting beneficial change. For either group of foundations, one issue is how optimal impact can be attained from successful, grant-funded innovations. If we look through the lens of grantmaking as investment, this issue can be cast as "optimizing return on investment."

The context, the reader will recall, is that foundations really have comparatively few resources and some, such as the Kellogg Foundation, invest these "at the margin" in innovation. How can the greatest benefit be gained from placing resources in this way? Return on investment is not measured simply in terms of whether, say, more people received services during the life of a grant – although this outcome is sought and measured by foundations – but whether, as a result of the project, more people will *continue* to receive services. In the particular case of the CBPH Initiative, the primary consideration was whether universities would continue to provide internal support to community-based teaching, research, and service and would maintain partnerships with health departments and CBOs.

Put simply, optimal impact from a successful, grant-funded innovation often will depend on whether change lasts, whether change spreads, and whether change is built on to achieve a higher order of change.

Will a grant-funded innovation be financially sustained through an ongoing funding stream (as opposed to a perpetual search for new grants)? Will it be institutionalized and become part of the way of doing business? Of course, innovations that are institutionalized may well be financially sustained by becoming part of ongoing operations. The innovation may be incorporated into operations in such a way that it is no longer recognizable as the "project," but has become part of other work. Nonetheless, financial sustainability and institutionalization are not identical.

Two developments have been going on simultaneously. At the same time that some grantmakers are more intentional about fostering the endurance of successful innovations, a number of evaluators have been addressing how change in communities occurs. If the developmental process by which change occurs can be well understood, then change efforts can be improved. The underlying concern for evaluators and grantmakers interested in communities is the same: the invest-

> *The greatest risk in making a social investment arises not because the undertaking may fail but because it may succeed.... A project may succeed brilliantly but prove to be grant-dependent and ultimately collapse.*

ment of time, money, and effort in ways that actually result in the solving of social problems.

Even successful innovations that are institutionalized and sustained for the project area and population may not lead to optimal return on investment. This is so for two reasons. First, the innovation may not be brought to scale. It may be preserved but only with the scope of a pilot project. It may not reach all those it might if the innovation were more broadly institutionalized and, further, incorporated into the networks of the organizations and groups involved. Next year, only a few blocks over, for example, in an area with essentially the same context another organization (even with some of the same partners) may "reinvent the wheel" with another innovation and tackle the same problem with a project. Or, in the same area, the next steps to keep the change-process progressing to the next stages, building on the successful innovation, are not taken. So, the successful innovation is preserved but it does not become the basis for an evolutionary change-process that can realize the full promise in the innovation.

The second reason a sustained successful innovation may not yield optimal return on investment from the perspective of actually solving social problems is that it may not be replicated by others in different locations and contexts. Fostering replication and implementing replication are both formidable tasks. Grantees – aside from being too busy to give much help – may not have appropriate skills for helping would-be replicators adapt a project to a different context. "Take away" documentation of project implementation may not be compiled in user-friendly form and may not even exist. Changeover in leadership or staffing of grant-funded projects is not uncommon and, by the time a would-be replicator appears on the scene, the institutional memory may be gone and with it the valuable explanation of what was essential and nonessential, and what worked and what flopped at the beginning. Even with good information and guidance about a good model that seems to "fit," would-be replicators cannot take shortcuts in building consensus and commitment in their own communities with respect to the approach to be replicated.

The Foundation's programming has been evolving for about a decade to greater and greater intentionality in meeting and managing risks. During the CBPH Initiative we were less experienced. When we announced to the grantees, well into the initiative, that they were to take on action planning to inform policy discussions, they were displeased, to say the least. Our reasoning was that informing policy could help to

achieve sustainability and institutionalization. We thought that integrating work on policy education, evaluation, and communications would make all three more effective. Our reasoning may have been good, but our timing was off. We introduced the concept of informing policy too late in the course of the initiative. The initiative evaluators concluded that pairing capacity building with goals for systems change and policy education is a significant challenge.

We have since gotten better, at least we think so. Today, we attempt to be explicit, timely, and supportive in recognizing both the challenge and the importance to grantees of integrating policy education into their work. We believe that change targets (with policy as an element of systems change) should be identified early in the design of an initiative – recognizing that the targets may be modified as the initiative matures. For example, in the **Community Voices: HeathCare for the Underserved** Initiative begun in 1998, we explicitly asked for identification of policy education targets in the proposals and we provide ongoing support for grantees' policy work through an intermediary. Despite the challenges, establishing policy objectives at the *beginning* of an initiative and developing and implementing strategies to educate policymakers throughout the process are both feasible and reflective of more recent Foundation grantmaking.

In addition to working on the policy targets they have identified, the Community Voices projects are expected to serve as learning laboratories. One focus of learning is internal, so that what is happening is reflected on and understood by those involved. A second focus is external so that people in other organizations and communities can learn and discern what elements of a project would work for them in their own locales.

The Turning Point Initiative uses a National Program Office, which is the National Association of County and City Health Officials (NACCHO), to support and work with grantees. In the process NACCHO is further developing its own capacity, which we anticipate will support dissemination, sustainability, maturation, and replication of Turning Point partnership models.

Creating a new entity to support sustainability, dissemination, policy education, and replication is another approach we are trying. The **Comprehensive Community Health Models of Michigan**, a major seven-year initiative, is now in transition as it closes. The operations office we created to help us manage the initiative has become the new independent **Center for Advancing Community Health**, part of the Michigan Public Health Institute.

These, then, are among the steps we have initiated to increase our ability to be a strategic risktaker who helps our grantees and the field gain optimal benefit from our investments.

# Conclusion

The Community-Based Public Health Initiative tested tripartite partnership as a means to revitalize public health professions education. The theory in the partnership model was that the agency and community partners would function as levers for change within the academic institutions. But, whichever end of the lever a partner was on, the partnership structure would give it new opportunities for change and growth in relationships with disparate partners. Overall, the CBPH Initiative seeded change in all three types of partners – academic, agency, and community. The Foundation's investment also leveraged other investments in CBPH. We invested $14 million and the projects raised an additional $25 million, or 180 percent of our investment.

With respect to sustainability, grantors and grantees face parallel tasks when an initiative is over. A grantee faces the task of sustaining the new way of doing business developed in the project. The grantor faces the task of sustaining in its programming what it has learned from the initiative. Both grantor and grantee have options for how to do their respective tasks. One of the interesting developments among the CBPH grantees' various efforts to sustain their new ways of doing business was the decision to work *across* sites. A partner at any one site would have quite a lot to do to maintain its own activities after the grant was over and even more to do to contribute to maintaining the site's CBPH consortium. For the grantees to attempt to maintain effort by collaborating across sites meant that, in some sense, they wanted to take on sustaining the *initiative* after funding had ended. This is uncommon in the grantmaking world, where most of the worry by grantee and grantor is about what will happen to the *project* after funding ends. Participants in CBPH created the **Center for the Advancement of Community Based Public Health**, which was their idea, although they applied for and received seed money from the Foundation. Through it they may perpetuate the legacy of CBPH by informing policy and practice and mobilizing widening participation in the CBPH principles. They were also instrumental in informing a CBPH caucus within the American Public Health Association.

The Kellogg Foundation has funded two programs, Turning Point: Collaborating for a New Century in Public Health and Community Health Scholars, to bring lessons learned from CBPH to the next stage of development and of capacity to inform ongoing and sustained change. Further, public health departments are central participants in several of the 13 sites in Community Voices: HealthCare for the Underserved, the six-year initiative to strengthen the delivery system and to increase coverage for the uninsured and access for the underserved.

This book demonstrates the commitment of its editors, authors, their colleagues, and organizations to sustained and widening community-oriented change in the field of public health. To the editors, authors, and you, the reader, we wish to express the Foundation's appreciation for the personal investments all are making to advance such change. While seen as independent and courted for their dollars, foundations are actually totally dependent on what others can accomplish. Foundations are background figures and risktakers; staff in foundations know where the action really is. For those, then, who are where the action is, this chapter has been written as a contribution to and appreciation of your effort.

# References

David R. *Community Voices: Challenges and Opportunities (What Has Love To Do With It?).* Keynote Address. Community Voices: HealthCare for the Underserved Meeting, Stowe, VT; August 1998.

Institute of Medicine. *The Future of Public Health.* Washington D.C.: National Academy of Sciences Press; 1988.

Kawachi I and Kennedy BP. Income inequality and health: Pathways and mechanisms. *Health Services Research.* 1999; 34(1):215-27.

Reis TK and Clohesy SJ. *Unleashing New Resources and Entrepreneurship for the Common Good: A Scan, Synthesis and Scenario for Action.* Battle Creek, MI: W.K. Kellogg Foundation; 1999.

# Appendix A | Community-Based Public Health Competencies

**Prepared by:** Faculty from Johns Hopkins University School of Public Health – Bone L; Geilen A; Shediac M; Johnson M; Farfel M; Burke T; Guyer B; Armenian H; and Zeger S.

## Preface

We would like to acknowledge the W.K. Kellogg Foundation's support for the Maryland Community-Based Public Health Initiative which made the development of the Community-Based Public Health Competencies possible. We appreciate the input, review, and comments from the Maryland Community-Based Public Health Initiative Partnership, East Baltimore Community residents, as well as the Washington University Community-Based Public Health Initiative and the University of California Berkeley School of Public Health/Oakland Community-Based Public Health Initiative.

## Community-Based Public Health Competencies

### Objective of Community-Based Public Health:

To provide Johns Hopkins Health Institutions[*] graduate students opportunities to learn the scope of community-based public health and the skills necessary to function in leadership roles in public agencies and community organizations.

### Background:

**Career Opportunities** – The education and training of public health professionals in community-based public health will prepare such individuals for careers which include, but are not limited to: primary medical care delivery (pediatrics, internal medicine, family practice) in a community setting, community health nursing and

community health education, as well as to prepare them for leadership roles in health departments or ministries of health, community health centers, voluntary associations, and other community-based organizations.

**Student Selection** – Students selecting this option would be early to mid-career professionals with an interest in and a commitment to community-based public health practice. Students would include physicians, nurses, health educators, community organizers, nutritionists, physical therapists, social workers, health care administrators, policy analysts, and epidemiologists.

**Community-Based Competencies** – The Community-Based Public Health Competencies that follow build upon the Schools of Public Health Faculty Agency Forum Competencies. It is recognized that significant basic knowledge related to illness and disease as well as health promotion are also necessary for public health students. The Community-Based Public Health Competencies are viewed as a supplement to the Public Health Faculty Agency Forum's Competencies, and are specific to health practice in the community setting. It is noteworthy that the new broad categories, Advocacy and Consultation, have been added. It is not anticipated that all of these competencies would be acquired upon completion of a graduate level degree program, but that the acquisition of such skills would be acquired and enhanced through a student's education, training, and professional experiences in public health practice.

**CBPH Application** – The Community-Based Public Health Competencies can be used to evaluate existing curricula and practicum and determine where gaps exist so that additional courses, and/or refocusing of existing courses, could take place. Field experiences, under skilled supervision, are recommended for the development of many of the suggested competencies. This will require formal linkages with local agencies and organizations and shared supervisory responsibility.

[*] Schools of Public Health, Medicine, and Nursing.

117

Faculty from health schools may need to be involved in these organizations as one component of their professional service. Preceptors/supervisors from the training site will need to be better integrated within our schools; for some this may mean instructional responsibility and a Faculty Associate position.

**Format:**

Listed in the first column in bold are the Faculty Agency Forum's Competencies. In *italics* in the second column are the Community-Based Public Health Competencies.

## Competencies

The Community-Based Public Health Competencies are the result of the deliberations of the Johns Hopkins School of Public Health's Working Group and discussions with members of the community, including leaders and volunteer activists as well.

| Faculty Agency Forum Public Health Competencies | Additional Competencies for Community-Based Public Health |
|---|---|

## 1. Analytic Skills

| | |
|---|---|
| • **Defining a problem.** | *Assessing community status: Developing community assessment skills; this involves: defining community and its sectors (e.g. political, economic, educational, religious), assessment of community health status and health needs, and assessment of community resources including: leadership, community organizations, etc. (Utilizing multidisciplinary perspective such as anthropological, sociological, psychological).* |
| | *Defining a problem, in conjunction with the community.* |
| | *Detecting and describing (using quantitative and qualitative data) infectious disease outbreaks, chronic disease clusters, and environmental risk factors.* |
| • **Understanding basic research designs used in public health.** | *Understanding appropriate research design and sampling approaches for community-based research.* |
| | *Understanding the balance between research and community needs.* |
| • **Determining appropriate use of data and statistical methods for problem identification and resolution, and program planning, implementation and evaluation.** | *Designing data collection instruments; collecting, evaluating and interpreting qualitative and quantitative data.* |
| | *Designing surveillance and monitoring systems.* |
| • **Selecting and defining variables relevant to defined public health problems.** | |

| Faculty Agency Forum Public Health Competencies | Additional Competencies for Community-Based Public Health |
|---|---|
| **1. Analytic Skills (Cont.)** | |
| • **Evaluating the integrity and comparability of data and identifying gaps in data sources.** | |
| • **Making relevant inferences from data.** | *Understanding appropriate statistical analyses for community-level and individual-level data.*<br><br>*Obtaining full community participation so that interpretations of inferences from the data reflect values and interpretation/understanding of the priorities and needs of the community.*<br><br>*Incorporate community perspective in every aspect of the process, including conceptualization, data instruments, and interpretation and dissemination of the results.* |
| • **Understanding how the data illuminate ethical, political, scientific, economic, and overall public health issues.** | |
| **2. Communication Skills** | |
| • **Communicating effectively both in writing and orally (unless a handicap precludes oral communication).** | *Being sensitive to local variations/dialects of language.*<br><br>*Developing public information and educational materials.*<br><br>*Determining how community gives and receives information (i.e., understanding different styles of communication and leadership).* |
| • **Presenting accurately and effectively demographic, statistical, programmatic, and scientific information for professional and lay audiences.** | *Presenting adequately and clearly the concepts of prevention and illness.*<br><br>*Explaining how public health relates to community health/primary care/personal care/self care.* |
| • **Soliciting input from individuals and organizations.** | *Understanding how to select and access key community leaders and informants in the community.*<br><br>*Applying community skills at the grassroots level.*<br><br>*Understanding how public health programs and agencies operate (e.g., Public Health infrastructure).* |
| • **Advocating for public health programs and resources.** | *Advocating for inclusion of target population or coalitions.* |

119

| Faculty Agency Forum<br>Public Health Competencies | Additional Competencies for<br>Community-Based Public Health |
|---|---|
| **2. Communication Skills (Cont.)**<br><br>• **Leading and participating in teams of individuals to address specific issues.** | *Participating and leading multi-disciplinary teams.*<br><br>*Advocating for inclusion of target individuals and coalitions.*<br><br>*Conducting effective meetings and utilizing formalized agreed upon governance structure (where appropriate).* |
| | *Understanding how to develop and maintain collaborative relationships and build coalitions.*<br><br>*Understanding how to negotiate and resolve conflicts.*<br><br>*Understanding how to develop and maintain multi-cultural teams utilizing group process skills in organizing, planning and development.*<br><br>*★ Fostering clear communication between health care providers and consumers.*<br><br>*★ Applying principles from relevant theories to communication strategies including, but not limited to: persuasive communication, diffusion, adult learning, social marketing and social action.*<br><br>*★ Interacting with the media to communicate important public health information.* |
| **3. Policy Development/ Program Planning Skills**<br><br>• **Collecting and summarizing data relevant to an issue in policy and program development, implementation and evaluation.** | |
| • **Identifying public health laws, regulations, and policies related to specific programs.** | *Understanding the structure and function of political/economic forces that influence government and policy.*<br><br>*Understanding the structure and function of government (e.g., legislative process).* |
| • **Stating policy options.** | *Articulating public health interventions based on community input and health status indicators.* |
| • **Stating the feasibility and expected outcomes of each policy option.** | *Understanding strategies for planned social change at micro and macro levels (e.g., individual health behaviors, normative environment, or organizational policy).* |

| Faculty Agency Forum<br>Public Health Competencies | Additional Competencies for<br>Community-Based Public Health |
|---|---|
| **3. Policy Development/ Program Planning Skills (Cont.)** | *Understanding the importance of community and citizen participation in social change efforts.*<br><br>*Developing flexible programs which enhance community competencies and ownership.* |
| • **Deciding on the appropriate course of action.** | |
| • **Writing a clear and concise policy statement.** | |
| • **Translating policy into organizational plans, structures, and programs** | |
| • **Developing a plan to implement policies, including goals, outcome and process objectives, and implementation steps.** | *Facilitating the community's leadership in the development of plan, selection of interventions, and implementation strategies.*<br><br>*Mastering a broad array of state-of-the-art intervention strategies and their effectiveness.*<br><br>*Understanding how to tailor interventions to meet the unique needs of different groups.* |
| • **Developing mechanisms to monitor and evaluate programs for their effectiveness and quality.** | *Applying methods for evaluating community-based programs.*<br><br>*Analyzing the cost-effectiveness and cost benefits of programs.*<br><br>*Implementing strategies to enhance program sustainability.*<br><br>*Identifying strategies to encourage replication and dissemination of effective programs.*<br><br>*Applying principles from relevant theories to program planning. Such theories include, but are not limited to: planned change, community development and social action.* |
| **4. Cultural Competencies** | |
| • **Understanding the dynamic forces contributing to cultural diversity.** | *Understanding the effect and manifestations of institutionalized oppression (racism, sexism, and classism) and how these forces impact the health of populations.* |

121

| Faculty Agency Forum<br>Public Health Competencies | Additional Competencies for<br>Community-Based Public Health |
|---|---|
| **4. Cultural Competencies (Cont.)** | |
| • **Interacting sensitively, effectively, and professionally with persons from diverse cultural, socioeconomic, educational, and professional backgrounds, and with persons of all ages and lifestyle preferences.** | |
| • **Identifying the role of cultural, social, environmental and behavioral factors in determining disease, disease prevention, health promoting behavior, and medical service.** | *Utilizing a broadly based framework which includes social, political, and economic perspectives in the development of community interventions.*<br><br>*Developing and adapting approaches to problems and materials that take into account cultural and language differences.* |
| **5. Basic Public Health Sciences Skills** | |
| • **Defining assessing, and understanding the health status of populations, determinants of health and illness, factors contributing to health promotion and disease prevention, and factors influencing the use of health services.** | *Understanding the communities' systems of health and healing.* |
| • **Applying the basic public health sciences including behavioral and social sciences, biostatistics, epidemiology, environmental public health, and prevention of chronic and infectious diseases and injuries.** | |
| • **Understanding the historical development and structure of state, local, and federal public health agencies.** | *Understanding the historical development and structure of communities.*<br><br>*Understanding the ethical and political issues in community-based research and service programs.* |

122

| Faculty Agency Forum<br>Public Health Competencies | Additional Competencies for<br>Community-Based Public Health |
|---|---|
| **6. Financial Planning and Management Skills** | |
| • **Developing and presenting a budget.** | *Understanding the political and economic forces that impact on the development of budget.* |
| • **Managing programs within budgetary constraints.** | |
| • **Developing strategies for determining budget priorities.** | |
| • **Monitoring program performance.** | |
| • **Preparing proposals for funding from external sources.** | *Developing joint proposals with community partners for fund-raising.* |
| • **Applying basic human relations skills for the internal management of organizations and for resolving internal and external conflicts.** | |
| • **Managing personnel.** | *Understanding how to maximize and coordinate human resources, including how to identify, train, supervise, and fund community residents to advocate and provide services.*<br><br>*Working with volunteers.*<br><br>*Building community infrastructure that enables the community to sustain current and initiate new programs.* |
| • **Understanding the theory of organizational structure and its influence upon professional work.** | |

123

| Faculty Agency Forum<br>Public Health Competencies | Additional Competencies for<br>Community–Based Public Health |
|---|---|
| | **7. Advocacy**<br><br>*Understanding how to negotiate and mediate.*<br><br>*Developing advocacy skills such as political consciousness-raising skills.*<br><br>*Understanding how to build constituencies and how to represent a constituency.*<br><br>*Understanding how to plan for and influence change.*<br><br><br>**8. Consultation**<br><br>*Providing training, consultation, and technical assistance to community groups in all competency areas.* |

124

# References From the Community-Based Public Health Initiative

Baker EA and Brownson CA. Defining characteristics of community-based health promotion programs. *Journal of Public Health Management and Practice*. 1998; 4:1-9.

Barnett K. *Collaboration for Community Empowerment: Re-defining the Role of Academic Institutions.* University of California School of Public Health, Berkeley: Center for Community Health; 1993.

Beilenson PL, Miola ES, Farmer M. Politics and practice: Introducing Norplant into a school-based health center in Baltimore. *American Journal of Public Health*. 1995; 85:309-11.

Brown L and Vega W. A protocol for community-based research. *American Journal of Preventive Medicine*. 1996; suppl. 12:4-5.

Brownson RC, Riley P, Bruce TA. Demonstration projects in community-based prevention. *Journal of Public Health Management and Practice*. 1998; 4:66-77 (also in *Topics in Community-Based Prevention*, edited by Lloyd F. Novick, Aspen Publishers; to be published).

Bruce TA. Educating policymakers and health planners. *American Journal of Preventive Medicine*. 1994; suppl. to 10:45-6.

Bruce TA. Public health principles in the regeneration of medical education. *Proceedings of World Summit on Medical Education,* Edinburgh. 1994; 28:68-70.

Bruce TA. Community health sciences: A discipline whose time has already come. *American Journal of Preventive Medicine*. 1995; suppl. to11:7.

Bruce TA. Medical education in community sites. *Medical Education*. 1996; 30:81-2.

Bruce TA and Uranga McKane S. Community-based public health. In CA Miller, P Halverson, and G Mays (eds.) *Book of Case Studies in Local Public Health Practice*. American Public Health Association Press; (in publication).

Bruce TA, Uranga McKane S, Grace HK. Community-based public health. *The University in the Urban Community: Responsibilities for Public Health*. Proceedings of the Sun Valley Forum on National Health, Association of Academic Health Centers; 1995.

Buchanan DR. Building academic-community linkages for health promotion: A case study in Massachusetts. *American Journal of Health Promotion*. 1996; 10:262-94.

Chen AM, Wismer BA, Lew R, Kang SH, Min K, Moksowitz JM, Tager IB. Health is strength: A research collaboration involving Korean Americans in Alameda County. *American Journal of Preventive Medicine*. 1997; 13:93-100.

Dual PA and Paroo IF. Urban health in the twenty-first century: The case for a community-based school of public health. *The University in the Urban Community: Responsibilities for Public Health*. Proceedings of the Sun Valley Forum on National Health, Association of Academic Health Centers; 1995.

Eng E, Parker E, Harlan C. Lay health advisor intervention strategies: A continuum from natural helping to paraprofessional helping. *Health Education and Behavior*. 1997; 24:413-7.

Evans CA. The role of city, county, and state health departments in the university-community interaction. *The University in the Urban Community: Responsibilities for Public Health*. Proceedings of the Sun Valley Forum on National Health, Association of Academic Health Centers; 1995.

Hill MN, Bone LR, Butz AM. Enhancing the role of community-health workers in research. *Journal of Nursing Scholarship*. 1996; 28:221-6.

Institute of Medicine. *Healthy Communities: New Partnerships for the Future of Public Health*. Washington, DC: National Academy Press; 1996.

Israel BA, Checkoway B, Schulz AJ, Zimmerman MA. Health education and community empowerment: Conceptualizing and measuring perceptions of individual, organizational, and community control. *Health Education Quarterly*. 1994; 21:149-70.

Israel BA, Cummings KM, Dignan MB, Heaney CA, Perales DP, Simons-Morton BG, Zimmerman MA. Evaluation of health education programs: Current assessment and future directions. *Health Education Quarterly*. 1995; 22:364-89.

Israel BA, Schulz AJ, Parker EA, Becker AB. Review of community-based research: Assessing partnership approaches to improve public health. *Annual Review of Public Health*. 1998.

Lashof JC. Building partnerships for healthy communities: The role of the academic health center. *American Journal of Public Health*. Editorial. 1994; 84:1070-1.

Levine DM, Becker DM, Bone LR. Narrowing the gap in health status of minority populations: A community-academic medical center partnership. *American Journal of Preventive Medicine*. 1992; 8:319-23.

Levine DM, Becker DM, Bone LR. A partnership with minority populations: A community model of effectiveness research. *Journal of Ethnicity and Disease*. 1992; 2:296-305.

Levine DM, Becker DM, Bone LR, Hill MN, Tuggle II MB, Zeger SL. Caring for the uninsured and underinsured: Community-academic health center partnerships for underserved minority populations. *Journal of the American Medical Association*. 1994; 272:309-11.

Milio N. *Engines of Empowerment: Using Information Technology to Create Healthy Communities and Challenge Public Policy*. Chicago, IL: Health Administration Press; 1996.

Omenn GS. The context for a future school of public health committed to urban health needs. *The University in the Urban Community: Responsibilities for Public Health*. Proceedings of the Sun Valley Forum on National Health, Association of Academic Health Centers; 1995.

Parker EA, Schulz AJ, Israel BA, Hollis RM. Detroit's East Side village health worker partnership: Community-based lay health advisor intervention in an urban area. *Health Education and Behavior*. 1998; 25:24-45.

Richardson WC, Field PM. The role of the university in urban health. *The University in the Urban Community: Responsibilities for Public Health*. Proceedings of the Sun Valley Forum on National Health, Association of Academic Health Centers; 1995.

Rowitz L. Reengineering public health: The two cultures revisited. *Journal of Public Health Management and Practice*. 1998; 4:78-80.

Schulz AJ, Israel BA, Becker AB, Hollis RM. "It's a twenty-four hour thing ... a living-for-each-other concept:" Identity, networks and community in an urban village health worker project. *Health Education & Behavior*. 1997; 24:465-80.

Schulz AJ, Parker EA, Israel BA, Becker AB, Maciak BJ, Hollis RM. Conducting a participatory community-based survey for a community health intervention on Detroit's East Side. *Journal of Public Health Management and Practice*. 1998; 4:10-24.

Shediac-Rizkallah MC, Bone LR. Planning for the sustainability of community-based health programs: Conceptual frameworks and future directions for research, practice, and policy. *Health Education Research*. 1998; 13:87-108.

Stillman FA, Bone LR, Rand C, Levine DM, Becker DM. Heart, Body, and Soul: A church-based smoking cessation program for urban African Americans. *Preventive Medicine*. 1993; 22:335-49.

Torres MI. Assessing health in an urban neighborhood: Community process, data results and implications for practice. *Journal of Community Health*. 1998; 23:211-26.

Uranga McKane S. Contexts for diversity. *Journal of Dental Education.* Reactions. 1995; 59:1119-22.

Voorhees CC, Stillman FA, Swank RT, Heagerty PJ, Levine DM, Becker DM. Heart, Body, and Soul: Impact of church-based smoking cessation interventions on readiness to quit. *Preventive Medicine.* 1996; 25:277-85.

## Special Reports

Auerbach M. Evaluation of the HEAP program of the Wake County Coalition. Master's thesis. School of Public Health, University of North Carolina, Chapel Hill; 1995.

Bruce TA. Community partnerships in health personnel education. Symposium report of a Problem-Based, Community-Centered, Learning Conference, Umtata, Transkei, South Africa; August 3, 1994.

Bruce TA. Around the world ... community health development: Report on the Salzburg Seminar. *CEDROS Network Newsletter,* Rio de Janeiro; June 1995.

Dixon T. Evaluation of canoe-pulling vs non-canoe-pulling. Graduate paper. School of Public Health and Community Medicine, University of Washington, Seattle; 1995.

Hegner R and Henderson RL. Community-based public health: A site vist to central North Carolina. *National Health Policy Forum Report;* May 31, 1995.

Neak R. Capacity of African-American communities: Results of a grounded theory study. Master's thesis. School of Public Health, University of North Carolina, Chapel Hill; 1995.

Werner KE and Clark NM. Meeting the public health challenges of a new era: Report of the School of Public Health Review Committee. University of Michigan, Ann Arbor; March 1994.

## Appendix C | Web Sites

The following are on-line addresses to learn more about W.K. Kellogg Foundation initiatives in community-based public health and health improvement and the work of other resource organizations.

Campus-Community Partnerships in Health:
**www.futurehealth.ucsf.edu/ccph.html**

Center for the Advancement of Community Based Public Health:
**www.cbph.org**

Coalition for Healthier Cities and Communities:
**www.healthycommunities.org**

Community-Based Public Health (CBPH) Initiative:
**www.wkkf.org/programminginterests/health/archive/626.htm**

Community Care Network National Demonstration of the Health Research and Educational Trust:
**www.aha.org/hret**

Community Health Scholars Program:
**www.sph.umich.edu/chsp**

Community Partnerships with Health Professions Education (CPHPE) Initiative:
**www.wkkf.org/programminginterests/health/archive/621.htm**

Community Voices: HealthCare for the Underserved:
**www.communityvoices.org**

Graduate Medical and Nursing Education (GMNE) Initiative:
**www.cpgmne.org**

National Program Office at the National Association for County and City Health Officials (NACCHO) for the Turning Point Initiative:
**www.naccho.org/project30.htm**

Turning Point: Collaborating for a New Century in Public Health:
**www.wkkf.org/programminginterests/health/TurningPoint/618.htm**

W.K. Kellogg Foundation:
**www.wkkf.org**

OVER RA 445 .C668 2000 c.1

Community-based public
  health

## DATE DUE